Atkins Diet Slow Cooker Cookbook

Prep -And-Go Simple And Flavored Recipes Made For Your Crock Pot To Rapid Weight Loss And Be More Healthier (Low Carb Diet, Ketogenic Diet, Keto Diet)

By Jennifer Hellen

© Copyright 2017- Jennifer Heller -All rights reserved.

In no way is it legal to reproduce, duplicate, or transmit any part of this document by either electronic means or in printed format. Recording of this publication is strictly prohibited, and any storage of this material is not allowed unless with written permission from the publisher. All rights reserved.

The information provided herein is stated to be truthful and consistent, in that any liability, regarding inattention or otherwise, by any usage or abuse of any policies, processes, or directions contained within is the solitary and complete responsibility of the recipient reader. Under no circumstances will any legal liability or blame be held against the publisher for any reparation, damages, or monetary loss due to the information herein, either directly or indirectly.

Legal Notice:
This book is copyright protected. This is only for personal use. You cannot amend, distribute, sell, use, quote or paraphrase any part or the content within this book without the consent of the author or copyright owner. Legal action will be pursued if this is breached.

Disclaimer Notice:
Please note the information contained within this document is for educational and entertainment purposes only. Every attempt has been made to provide accurate, up to date and reliable, complete information. No warranties of any kind are expressed or implied. Readers acknowledge that the author is not engaging in the rendering of legal, financial, medical or professional advice.

By reading this document, the reader agrees that under no circumstances are we responsible for any losses, direct or indirect, which are incurred as a result of the use of information contained within this document, including, but not limited to, — errors, omissions, or inaccuracies.

Table of Contents

Introduction 5

Chapter 1: Essentials of Atkins Diet 6

What is the Atkins diet? 6

The History of Atkins Diet 6

How Does It Work? 7

Why it is Effective for Weight Loss? 7

The Benefits of the Atkins Diet 8

Chapter 2: Atkins Diet Plan 10

Atkins Diet Step-by-Step 10

    Phase 1: Induction 10

    Phase 2: Balancing 12

    Phase 3: Fine Tuning 13

    Phase 4: Maintenance 14

Chapter 3: Atkins Grocery-shopping Guide 16

What Groceries Will I Need to Get Started? 16

What Can I Eat? 18

    Phase 1: 18

    Phase 2 22

    Phase 3 23

    Phase 4 25

What Should I Avoid? 26

Chapter 4: Using a Slow Cooker on Atkins Diet 28

What is Slow Cooking? 28

Benefits of Slow Cooking 28

FAQs of Slow Cooking 29

30 Easy-to-Follow Slow Cooker Recipes for the Atkins Diet 31

- 1. Simple and Delicious Chicken Enchiladas 32
- 2. Easy Heart-Warming Caramel Rolls 34
- 3. Unforgettable Slow-Cooker Tater Tots 36
- 4. Delicious Sausage and Egg Casserole 38
- 5. Tempting Breakfast Casserole with Tomato and Spinach 40
- 6. Scrumptious Breakfast Pie 42
- 7. Tender Autumn Oxtail Stew 44
- 8. Delicious Slow Cooked Poached Salmon 46
- 9. Delicious Slow-cooked Italian Beef 48
- 10. Mouthwatering Chicken and Kale Soup 50
- 11. Appetizing Orange Chicken 52
- 12. Delightful Garlic Butter Chicken with Cream Cheese Sauce 54
- 13. Slow-cooked Brats 56
- 14. Creamy Reuben Soup 58
- 15. Tasty Slow-cooked Pesto Chicken Salad 60
- 16. Delicious Stuffed Poblano Peppers 62
- 17. Yummy Cheesy Roasted Brussels dip 64
- 18. Heavenly Braised Cabbage 66

20. Slow Cooker Jerk Chicken..70

21. Slow Cooker Frittata...72

22. Tasty Tarragon Lamb Shanks with Cannellini Beans..................74

23. Delightful Carnitas & Paleo Nachos...76

24. Chicken Fajita Soup..78

25. Slow-Cooker Lemon and Olive Chicken.......................................80

26. Satisfying Pork Stew...82

27. Low-carb Slow-cooked Pizza..84

28. Easy Italian Zucchini Meatloaf...86

29. Hearty Beef Stew...88

30. Easy Slow-cooker Chicken Roast...90

FAQs..92

Can I drink alcohol or coffee on the Atkins Diet?.............................92

Can you drink soda and juices on the Atkins Diet?...........................92

How much weight can I lose by following the Atkins Diet?............92

Is this diet suitable for PCOS patients?...93

Is this diet suitable for diabetics?...93

Is the Atkins Diet compatible with veganism?....................................93

How can I ensure a nutritionally balanced diet when on Atkins?......93

Conclusion..95

Introduction

The Atkins diet is ideal for people who are struggling to lose some weight. While there are countless diet plans floating around on the internet that claim to help with weight loss, the Atkins diet is backed with scientific research. This cookbook will guide you through your journey towards a healthy body and help you achieve your goals. It will help you understand what exactly the Atkins diet is, and how it works to benefit your body.

There are four phases you will go through while following the Atkins diet. With this cookbook, you will learn about each phase and its respective diet plan. Along with this information, this cookbook will also help you understand the changes you'll be making in your lifestyle, and will guide you through the little tips and tricks that make a difference.

The Atkins Diet involves and encourages a lot of slow cooking. Wondering why exactly you should slow-cook your meals? Don't fret; this cookbook will explain all of the benefits that make slow cooking such an essential part of the Atkins diet. There are 30 easy-to-follow slow cooker recipes. A variety of recipes are included, covering soup, meat, vegetable, dessert, etc..

If you still have questions regarding the diet, the Frequently Asked Questions should have the answers you were looking for. The Atkins Diet might seem like a long and tough journey, but with proper guidance and support, you'll find what you've been looking for and fulfill your desired goals.

Chapter 1 Essentials of Atkins Diet

What is the Atkins diet?

Simply put, the Atkins diet is a low-carb, high-protein and high-fat diet. It's designed to help people struggling to lose weight and achieve their body goals. Followed properly, the Atkins diet is part of a healthy lifestyle.

The History of Atkins Diet

The Atkins Diet was developed in the early 1970's by a cardiologist named Robert C. Atkins, and it quickly gained a large following. Diets were common in the early 20th century, but all of the popular diets were temporary "quick fixes" based on deprivation or bizarre food choices. They focused on net calories per meal, instead of on the holistic notion of a permanent change to one's way of eating. Dr. Atkins was one of the first proponents of the idea that weight loss could be part of a healthy, sustainable lifestyle. The Atkins Diet is also backed by multiple scientific studies.

How Does It Work?

People's bodies respond differently to different stimuli; some people require a higher protein intake, while others do better when limiting carb intake. What the Atkins Diet does is allow each person to determine what type of food suits them and their metabolism.

There are two types of energy sources the body can use: sugar and fats. It's important to understand that the particular type of fuel you burn will affect how you lose weight and whether you can maintain the weight loss or not. Regular diets are focused solely on reducing calorie intake, but they don't account for the amount or proportion of fats, protein and carbohydrates that you consume.

Many years' worth of research has shown that the Atkins Diet is a safe and effective way to lose body fat and then maintain your desired weight level for as long as the plan is followed, which is not hard to do if you approach the diet knowing that it represents long-term change for you and your body.

Why it is Effective for Weight Loss?

When you eat, your body turns the carbohydrates in your food into sugar, specifically glucose, during digestion. Your metabolism runs on glucose, so your body likes to keep a 24-hour supply on hand, in the form of glycogen. Glycogen is your body's fuel source of choice. If you don't use your entire supply of glycogen within 24 hours, the unused glycogen will be deposited within your body as fat, and a new glycogen supply will be drawn from the food you consume. It's a constant cycle.

Unless your glycogen supply is exhausted, your body will not burn fat. Fat is your body's long-term energy storage solution; it's what keeps you alive when there's no food available, like during a famine. Your body has evolved to maintain fat storage for the sake of survival.

What all this means is that a high carbohydrate intake will keep your glycogen stores constantly full, which will prevent your body from burning fat, despite your best efforts with diet and exercise. The Atkins Diet helps you solve this problem in the following ways:

1. By reducing your daily carbohydrate intake, you will run through your glycogen stores more quickly and cause your body to burn more fat for energy. This not only helps in reducing the overall fat content of the body, but also ensures that the limited amount of carbohydrates taken in by the body are not left unused and converted to fat.

2. Since your calorie intake remains roughly the same, you shouldn't struggle with hunger or feeling deprived. Your body gets a stable source of energy- but just enough energy instead of too much. You should still feel energetic and satisfied, while you continue to lose weight. You may even find that foods recommended for the Atkins Diet are not that different from foods in your regular diet before.

3. You can customize the Atkins Diet for your specific needs, and that flexibility is what makes the Atkins Diet so sustainable for long-term change.

The Benefits of the Atkins Diet

The Atkins Diet delivers a considerable number of benefits, including:

1. Promoting effective weight loss;
2. Providing an understanding of your bodily needs;
3. Helping to decide which foods are best for your body;
4. Helping to maintain energy levels throughout the day;
5. Helping to avoid hunger-related temptations;
6. Allowing you to sustain a long-term healthy lifestyle .

Chapter 2 Atkins Diet Plan

Atkins Diet Step-by-Step

The Atkins Diet is a low-carb diet and is often recommended for those who want to lose weight, while still eating the same amount of protein and fats as before, but reducing carb intake. Low-carb diets have proven to be effective at reducing weight and the Atkins Diet is one of the most reputable forms of the low-carb diet. Here is a description of the Atkins 20 Diet:

Phase 1: Induction

The purpose of the induction phase is to introduce your body to fat-burning mode. The goal is to drop your daily carb intake the current level all the way down to an average of 20 grams (18 grams minimum, and 22 maximum) daily. This will lead to a smaller daily glycogen supply, which will allow the body to start burning fats earlier in the day once the glycogen is used up. This phase will last at least two weeks, though if you wish to burn more fat, you may continue for longer periods of time without a problem. Either way, you'll continue this phase until you are 15 pounds away from your goal. Here are some tips for eating in the induction phase:

- Eat three meals and two snacks a day, or even six small meals a day. The goal is to avoid becoming so hungry that you eat whatever is on hand; you want to eat each meal intentionally. Don't go more than three or four waking hours without eating.

- Consume 20 grams of Net Carbohydrates (NC) a day. Make sure most of these come from vegetables; about 12 – 15 grams.
- Make sure to include protein with every meal. You need protein to develop muscle mass, which will help with weight loss because muscle mass burns calories even at rest. In Phase 1, the recommendation is to consume three 4 – 6-ounce servings each day.
- Don't restrict your fat intake. Fats are important for many reasons; they help to make you feel full after eating a meal, contribute to the flavor of foods, and help your body absorb certain vitamins. Fat intake is crucial to the Atkins Diet.
- Drink at least eight 8-ounce servings of water throughout the day. This accounts for your entire fluid intake, so two of your "water" servings can be coffee or tea, and another two can be beef, chicken, or vegetable broth.
- You will initially experience some water loss; this is normal, but make sure to avoid dehydration or electrolyte imbalance. Helpful sources of sodium include salty broth, table salt, and soy sauce.
- Use sugar substitutes in moderation; three packets a day at most.
- Use only Atkins products where possible, since they have been tested to ensure minimal impact on your blood sugar level. Almost all Atkins products are suitable for Phase 1. Make sure that the remaining 5 – 8 grams of your daily carbohydrates come from either Atkins products, dairy or dressings (the rest being from vegetables).

You can enjoy some slow-cooked Italian beef or poached salmon during this phase.

Phase 2: Balancing

The purpose of this phase is to start transitioning from weight loss to maintenance, by find a balance of carbohydrates in your diet. Start at 25 grams daily, and raise your intake in 5-gram steps. Depending on a variety of factors, including but not limited to age, gender, activity level and/or hormonal status, your carb level can balance out at 30 – 80 grams a day. This phase continues until you are 10 pounds away from your goal weight. However, you can move to Phase 3 earlier; your weight loss will continue but at a slower rate compared to Phase 2. Here are some tips for eating in Phase 2:

- Continue to consume a minimum of 12–15 daily grams of Net Carbohydrates as vegetables. This Phase 1 rule is continued into Phase 2. Vegetables are rich in fiber and have the type of carbohydrates your body really needs. They are crucial to the Atkins diet.
- Follow a "carb ladder" and reintroduce foods to your diet one at a time. The intervals of adding foods may vary depending on your metabolism and weight-loss goal. You might follow weekly intervals, biweekly intervals or even longer.
- Add carbs back to your diet with each step of the ladder, one by one. For example, when you reintroduce one carb-heavy food, gauge the impact, if any, before reintroducing another one.
- Increase your overall daily Net Carb intake. Use no more than 5-gram increments on a weekly, bi-weekly or monthly interval.
- You will likely experience plateaus: times when you don't see much progress with regards to weight loss. If this happens, first double-check that you're doing everything correctly. If you are, and still not seeing the differences you want to see, it is recommended to add a bit of exercise to your routine.

Chicken and Kale soup is one of the most delicious dishes you can enjoy during this phase.

Phase 3: Fine Tuning

The purpose of this phase is to lose the last of your excess weight and further explore your carb balance; in this phase, you will find your ideal daily carb intake to maintain your weight. This phase is often considered preparation for lifelong weight maintenance. The goal here is to steadily increase your daily net carb intake in 10-gram steps, and to continue to reintroduce new carb-heavy foods so long as your weight is maintained. This phase will last till you have reached your goal weight and then afterwards, for another month of maintaining that weight. Here are some tips for eating in the fine-tuning phase:

- If You Hit a Plateau: As in Phase 2, first double-check that you're doing everything correctly; it's easy to get complacent and start to let things slip over time. If you are following the diet correctly and still not seeing progress, decrease your daily Net Carb intake by 10 grams and monitor for signs of progress.
- Finding Net Carb Tolerance: It is possible to stumble upon your Net Carb tolerance for weight maintenance in Phase 3; if you do, it might initially look like a plateau. Decrease 10 grams of your daily Net Carbohydrates for at least a week to see if this is the case. If weight loss resumes, go up another 5 grams, and so forth.

Enjoy some braised cabbage while you're in this phase. You can go through the recipes in this book to treat yourself with dishes that perfectly follow the Atkins Diet.

Phase 4: Maintenance

The purpose of this phase is to transition to a permanent weight-maintaining lifestyle. The goal here is to control your weight in case your carb tolerance changes, or if you gain some extra weight. This phase lasts indefinitely. If you are willing to adopt Phase 4 as a new lifestyle, then you may never need to diet again, since you now understand your bodily needs and compatibility with different types of foods. You have gone through the Atkins diet phase-by-phase, and have gradually developed a sustainable, healthy way of eating. Since you added foods back one at a time, you already know their effects, if any, on your body weight (regardless of whether those effects were permanent or not). You now understand which foods are best for maintaining your weight. You should also how to handle your cravings, how to substitute certain low-carb foods for high-carb ones, and how to enjoy other foods sparingly, as garnishes or finishing touches. Here is a tip for eating in the maintenance phase:

- If you have gained a few pounds, no problem; just cut roughly 10 grams of Net Carbohydrates a day from your intake until you return to your goal weight.

Travel Tips for Atkins Dieters:

1) Check if you will have access to a refrigerator during your stay, and stock up on Atkins-approved snacks.
2) If you know the restaurants where you'll be dining, check out the menu in advance to pre-select your low-carb options. Having a plan before you go out to eat makes it easier resist any high-carb temptations.
3) Try to stick with your usual meal schedule.

4) Inquire about what is in the dishes you are served, both at home and while eating out.
5) Eat only until you feel satisfied, not stuffed.
6) Drink alcohol in moderation if you are past the first phase of Atkins, and watch out for drinks containing sugar or fruit juice.
7) If your host pressures you to try something like cake or pie, politely decline by saying you're full, or eat a very small amount.
8) Offer to bring a low-carb option when attending an event in someone else's home.
9) Stay hydrated. Keep a water bottle with you and refill it frequently.
10) Stay active. Go for walks and try joining a gym or working out regularly.

Chapter 3 Atkins Grocery-shopping Guide

What Groceries Will I Need to Get Started?

When starting out on the Atkins diet, there are some items you will need to stock up on, especially in Phase 1. Below is a list of groceries to buy when following the Atkins diet.

Vegetables are a key part of Phase 1 of the Atkins Diet; you should be getting approximately 12 to 15 grams of Net Carbohydrates per day from vegetables. Once you hit Phase 2, you'll be allowed to incorporate certain fruits.

Salad Bases

- Romaine lettuce, Iceberg lettuce
- Arugula, Spinach, Endive

Snacks

- Celery, Cucumber, Bell Peppers

Salad Toppers

- Mushrooms, Avocadoes, Artichokes
- Radicchio, Radishes

Meat: All meat is allowed during all phases of Atkins. Here are some ideas:

- Bacon, Beef, Ham, Lamb, Pork

Poultry

- Chicken, Cornish Hen, Duck, Turkey

Seafood: All fish and shellfish are allowed in all phases of Atkins. Here are some ideas:

Fish

- Salmon, Tuna, Trout
- Cod, Halibut, Shellfish

Clams

- Crabmeat, Mussels, Oysters, Shrimp

Dairy

- Sour Cream, Mayonnaise

Cheese: The following cheeses are allowed in all phases of Atkins:

- Bleu , Cheddar , Goat , Cream Cheese
- Feta , American Cheese, Gouda
- Mozzarella, Parmesan, Swiss

Refrigerator Staples

- Eggs, Salad Dressings
- Lemon Juice, Lime Juice

Pantry Staples

- Chicken or Vegetable Broth or Bouillon Cubes, Splenda, Vegetable Oil
- Olive Oil, Herbs and Spices

Beverages

- Flavored Zero-Calorie Seltzer Water
- Diet Soda, Club Soda, Coffee, Tea

What Can I Eat?

Each of the four phases of the Atkins diet has its own food requirements. Here is a breakdown of acceptable foods at each phase of the Atkins diet:

Phase 1:

Foundation Vegetables	SERVING SIZE	NET CARBS
Alfalfa sprouts (raw)	1/2 cup	0
Chicory greens (raw)	1/2 cup	.1
Endive (raw)	1/2 cup	.1
Escarole (raw)	1/2 cup	.1
Olives, green	5, each	.1
Watercress (raw)	1/2 cup	.1
Arugula (raw)	1/2 cup	.2
Radishes (raw)	1, each	.2
Spinach (raw)	1/2 cup	.2
Bok choy (cooked)	1/2 cup	.4
Lettuce, average (raw)	1/2 cup	.5
Turnip greens (cooked)	1/2 cup	.6
Heart of palm	1 each	.7
Beet greens (cooked)	1/2 cup	1.8
Olives, black	5, each	.7
Radicchio (raw)	1/2 cup	.7
Asparagus (cooked)	6 stalks	1.9
Eggplant (cooked)	1/2 cup	2.3
Sprouts, mung beans (raw)	1/2 cup	2.2
Button mushrooms (raw)	1/2 cup	.8
Artichoke (marinated)	1, each	1
Celery (raw)	1 stalk	1
Collard greens (cooked)	1/2 cup	1
Pickle, dill	1, each	1
Broccoli (cooked)	1/2 cup	1.8
Rhubarb (raw)	1/2 cup	1.8
Cucumber, sliced (raw)	1/2 cup	1.6
Spinach	1/2 cup	1
Broccoli rabe (cooked)	1/2 cup	1.2
Sauerkraut (drained)	1/2 cup	1.2
Avocado, Haas	1/2 fruit	1.3

Daikon radish, grated (raw)	1/2 cup	1.4
Red/white onion, chopped (raw)	2 TBSP	1.5
Zucchini (cooked)	1/2 cup	1.5
Cauliflower (cooked)	1/2 cup	1.7
Fennel (raw)	1/2 cup	1.8
Okra (cooked)	1/2 cup	1.8
Swiss chard (cooked)	1/2 cup	1.8
Broccoli (cooked)	3, each	1.9
Bell pepper, green, chopped (raw)	1/2 cup	2.2
Kale (cooked)	1/2 cup	2.4
Green beans (cooked)	1/2 cup	2.9
Jicama (raw)	1/2 cup	2.6
Cherry tomato	10, each	4.6
Scallions, chopped (raw)	1/2 cup	2.4
Turnip (cooked)	1/2 cup	2.4
Tomato, small (raw)	1, each	2.5
Portobello mushroom (cooked)	1, each	2.6
Kohlrabi (cooked)	1/2 cup	4.6
Brussel sprouts (cooked)	1/2 cup	3.5
Leeks (cooked)	2 TBSP	3.4
Tomato (cooked)	1/2 cup	8.6
Garlic, minced (raw)	2 TBSP	5.3
Cabbage (cooked)	1/2 cup	2.7
Pumpkin, mashed (cooked)	1/2 cup	4.7
Spaghetti squash (cooked)	1/2 cup	4
Yellow squash (cooked)	1/2 cup	2.6
Bell pepper, red, chopped (raw)	1/2 cup	3
Shallot, chopped (raw)	2 TBSP	3.4
Snow peas (cooked)	1/2 cup	5.4

Approximately 12 to 15 grams of Net Carbohydrates per day should be consumed from vegetables. Depending on the actual carb content, this is equal to several cups of the desired vegetable, where a cup is roughly the size of a baseball. Measure salad vegetables raw.

Salad Garnishes	SERVING SIZE	NET CARBS
Crumbled bacon	3 slices	0
Hard-boiled egg	1 egg	.5
Sautéed mushrooms	1/2 cup	1.0
Sour cream	2 Tbsp.	1.2

Salad Dressings	SERVING SIZE	NET CARBS
Red wine vinegar	1 TBSP	0
Caesar	2 TBSP	1
Ranch	2 TBSP	1.4
Lemon juice	2 TBSP	2.0
Bleu cheese	2 TBSP	2.3

	SERVING SIZE	NET CARBS
Lime juice	2 TBSP	2.4
Balsamic vinegar	1 TBSP	2.7
Italian, creamy	2 TBSP	3

An acceptable salad dressing should have no added sugar and no more than 2 grams of Net Carbohydrates per serving (1-2 Tbsp)

Herbs and Spices	SERVING SIZE	NET CARBS
Basil	1 TBSP	0
Cayenne pepper	1 TBSP	0
Cilantro	1 TBSP	0
Dill	1 TBSP	0
Oregano	1 TBSP	0
Tarragon	1 TBSP	0
Parsley	1 TBSP	.1
Chives (fresh or dehydrated)	1 TBSP	.1
Ginger, fresh, grated	1 TBSP	.8
Rosemary, dried	1 TBSP	.8
Sage, ground	1 TSP	.8
Black pepper	1 TSP	.9
Garlic	1 clove	.9

Make sure herbs and spices contain no added sugar.

All Fish Including:
- Sole, Tuna, Trout
- Cod, Flounder
- Herring, Salmon
- Sardines
- Halibut

All Shellfish Including:
- Clams
- Oysters*
- Shrimp
- Squid
- Crabmeat
- Mussels*
- Lobster

*No more than 4 ounces of oysters and mussels per day, due to their high carb counts.

All Meat Including:
- Ham*
- Lamb, Pork
- Bacon*
- Beef, Veal
- Venison

*Some meats will add to your carb count; these include processed meats such as bacon and

sugar-cured ham. If possible, it is preferable to avoid meats with added nitrates, such as cold cuts.
All Poultry Including: • Chicken, Duck • Goose, Pheasant • Cornish hen • Quail, Turkey • Ostrich
Eggs in Any Style, Including: • Hard-boiled • Deviled, Scrambled • Fried, Omelette • Poached, Soft-boiled
Eggs are a staple breakfast in the Atkins Nutritional Approach, due to their high nutritional value. A little creativity can do wonders for your egg-based breakfasts and snacks: add onions, mushrooms or green pepper. A topping of feta cheese, basil, oregano and other herbs can also add variation.

Fats and Oils
1. Mayonnaise – with no added sugar
2. Olive oil
3. Butter
4. Vegetable oils – Olive oil is one of the best, but varieties that are expeller-pressed or cold-pressed are also very good.
    • Sesame
    • Walnut
    • Sunflower*
    • Safflower*
    • Canola*
    • Soybean*
    • Grape seed*

*it is best to not let the temperature of these oils get too high. Olive oil should be used for sautéing only. Walnut and sesame oil should be used only for dressing cooked vegetables or salad.

Cheese	SERVING SIZE	NET CARBS
Parmesan, grated	1 Tbsp.	.2
Goat or chèvre	1 oz.	.3
Bleu cheeses	2 Tbsp.	.4
Cheddar	1 oz.	.4
Gouda	1 oz.	.6
Mozzarella, whole milk	1 oz.	.6
Cream cheese, whipped	2 Tbsp.	.8
Parmesan, chunk	1 oz.	.9

Swiss	1 oz.	1.0
Feta	1 oz.	1.2

It is worth noting that cheese does contain about 1 gram per ounce of carbohydrates. Eat no more than 3-4 ounces of cheese per day. An ounce is almost the size of an individually-wrapped slice of cheese or a 1" cube.

Beverages
- Bouillon/Clear broth (no added sugar)
- Diet soda (note the carb count)
- Flavored seltzer (zero calorie)
- Cream, heavy or light
- Herbal tea (no fruit sugar or barley added)
- Unflavored soy/almond milk
- Decaffeinated or regular coffee and tea*
- Club soda
- Water – at least 8-ounce glasses per day including:
   Filtered water, Mineral water, Tap water, Spring water

* An individual may have one or two cups of coffee or caffeinated tea daily, according to their preference. Do not consume caffeine if symptoms of hypoglycemia or cravings are experienced as a result. The induction phase is best for breaking a caffeine addiction, should you suffer from one.

* Consume no more than 3 T of lemon and lime juices per day

* Consume no more than 3 TBSP or 1.5 fl. Oz. of cream (heavy or light) per day

Artificial Sweeteners
   Sucralose, saccharine or stevia – one packet equals 1 gram of Net Carbohydrates

** If you have decided to stay in the Induction phase longer than 2 weeks, you may swap out 3g NC of other foundation vegetables for 3g NC of nuts or seeds. Do not let your Foundation Vegetable levels drop below 12g NC.

Phase 2

Dairy	SERVING SIZE	NET CARBS
Mozzarella cheese	5 ounces	3.0
Yogurt, Greek	1/2 cup or 4 ounces	3.5
Ricotta cheese	1/2 cup	3.8
Cottage cheese, 2%	1/2 cup	4.1
Heavy cream	3/4 cup	4.8
Yogurt, Plain	1/2 cup or 4 ounces	5.5
Legumes (Cooked/Canned)	SERVING SIZE	NET CARBS
Lentils	1/4 cup	4
Kidney Beans	1/4 cup	5.9
Lima Beans	1/4 cup	6.1
Pinto Beans	1/4 cup	6.1
Black Beans	1/4 cup	6.5

Navy Beans	1/4 cup	10.1
Great Northern Beans	1/4 cup	10.6
Chickpeas	1/4 cup	10.9
Fruits	**SERVING SIZE**	**NET CARBS**
Blackberries (fresh)	1/4 cup	1.6
Raspberries (fresh)	1/4 cup	1.7
Cranberries (fresh)	1/4 cup	1.9
Strawberries, sliced (fresh)	1/4 cup	2.4
Cantaloupe, cubes	1/4 cup	2.9
Honeydew, cubes	1/4 cup	3.5
Gooseberries (fresh)	1/4 cup	3.9
Boysenberries (fresh)	1/4 cup	4.5
Blueberries (fresh)	1/4 cup	4.5
Juices	**SERVING SIZE**	**NET CARBS**
Lemon juice	2 TBSP	2.0
Lime juice	2 TBSP	2.4
Tomato juice	4 ounces	4.0
Nuts & Seeds (and Butters)	**SERVING SIZE**	**NET CARBS**
Brazil nuts	6 nuts	1.4
Macadamias	10 nuts	1.4
Hulled sunflower seeds	2 TBSP	1.5
Walnuts	12 nuts	1.7
Almonds	24 nuts	2.2
Pistachios	2 TBSP	3.0
Peanuts	2 TBSP	3.8
Pecans	2 TBSP	3.8
Cashews	2 TBSP	5.1
Convenience Foods		
Many of the foods listed above are available in convenient "snack-size" packaging at the supermarket or convenience store; feel free to grab and go – just note the serving size, and subtract the fiber from total carbohydrates to get the total Net Carbohydrates. Remember, Atkins bars and shakes are super convenient too, and every single flavor is allowed in Phase 2. So be busy, be happy and be well fed!		

Phase 3

Grains*	**SERVING SIZE**	**NET CARBS**
Wheat bran (raw)	2 TBSP	1.6
Wheat germ	2 TBSP	4.9
Oat bran (raw)	2 TBSP	6.0
Quinoa (cooked)	1/4 cup	8.6
Whole wheat bread	1 slice	10
Oatmeal (dry, steel cut)	1/4 cup	11.5
Polenta (dry)	2 TBSP	12.5

Grits (cooked)	1/2 cup	15.2
Whole wheat pasta (cooked)	1/2 cup	16.6
Oatmeal (dry, rolled)	1/3 cup	19
Barley (cooked)	1/2 cup	19.2
Millet (cooked)	1/2 cup	19.5
Rice (brown, cooked)	1/2 cup	21.2

* Be sure to check the nutrition label for the most current NC count. Individual brands may vary.

Starchy Vegetables*	**SERVING SIZE**	**NET CARBS**
Carrots, sliced	1 medium	4.1
Rutabaga, cubed	1/2 cup	5.9
Beets, sliced	1/2 cup	6.8
Peas	1/2 cup	7
Acorn Squash (baked/mashed)	1/2 cup	7.6
Butternut squash	1/2 cup	8.5
Sweet potato, baked	1/2 medium	9.9
Parsnips, sliced	1/2 cup	10.2
Potato, baked	1/2 small	13.1
Corn	1/2 cup	14.9

Fruit	**SERVING SIZE**	**NET CARBS**
Coconut, fresh, shredded	1/2 cup	2.5
Figs, fresh	1 fruit	4.5
Cherries	1/4 cup	5.3
Watermelon, cubes	1/2 cup	5.5
Pomegranate seeds	1/4 cup	6.4
Papaya, pieces	1/2 cup	6.6
Plum, medium	1 fruit	6.6
Guava	1/2 cup	7.4
Clementine	1 fruit	7.6
Apple	1/2 fruit	7.9
Kiwi	1 fruit	8.1
Grapefruit (red)	1/2 fruit	8.9
Apricot, medium	3 fruits	9.6
Pineapple, fresh, chunks	1/2 cup	9.7
Peach, small	1 fruit	10.5
Mango	1/2 cup	11.1
Grapes (red)	1/2 cup	13
Orange, navel	1 fruit	14.5
Dates, fresh	3 fruits	15.8
Banana, small	1 fruit	20.4
Pear, medium	1 fruit	21

* All figures are for cooked (not raw) vegetables, legumes, or grains.

Phase 4

Grains	SERVING SIZE	NET CARBS
Wheat bran (raw)	2 TBSP	1.6
Wheat germ	2 TBSP	4.9
Oat bran (raw)	2 TBSP	6.0
Quinoa (cooked)	1/4 cup	8.6
Whole wheat bread	1 slice	10
Oatmeal (dry, steel cut)	1/4 cup	11.5
Polenta (dry)	2 TBSP	12.5
Grits (cooked)	1/2 cup	15.2
Whole wheat pasta (cooked)	1/2 cup	16.6
Oatmeal (dry, rolled)	1/3 cup	19
Barley (cooked)	1/2 cup	19.2
Millet (cooked)	1/2 cup	19.5
Rice (brown, cooked)	1/2 cup	21.2

* Be sure to check the nutrition label for the most current NC count. Individual brands may vary.

Starchy Vegetables	SERVING SIZE	NET CARBS
Carrots, sliced	1 medium	4.1
Rutabaga, sliced	1/2 cup	5.9
Beets, sliced	1/2 cup	6.8
Peas	1/2 cup	7
Acorn squash (cubed/mashed)	1/2 cup	7.6
Butternut squash	1/2 cup	8.5
Sweet potato, baked	1/2 medium	9.9
Parsnips, sliced	1/2 cup	10.2
Potato, baked	1/2 small	13.1
Corn	1/2 cup	14.9

Fruit	SERVING SIZE	NET CARBS
Coconut, fresh, shredded	1/2 cup	2.5
Figs, fresh	1 fruit	4.5
Cherries	1/4 cup	5.3
Watermelon, cubes	1/2 cup	5.5
Pomegranate seeds	1/4 cup	6.4
Papaya, pieces	1/2 cup	6.6
Plum, medium	1 fruit	6.6
Guava	1/2 cup	7.4
Clementine	1 fruit	7.6
Apple	1/2 fruit	7.9
Kiwi	1 fruit	8.1
Grapefruit (red)	1/2 fruit	8.9
Apricot, medium	3 fruits	9.6

Pineapple, fresh, chunks	1/2 cup	9.7
Peach, small	1 fruit	10.5
Mango	1/2 cup	11.1
Grapes (red)	1/2 cup	13
Orange, navel	1 fruit	14.5
Dates, fresh	3 fruits	15.8
Banana, small	1 fruit	20.4
Pear, medium	1 fruit	21

What Should I Avoid?

Foods other than those listed above are to be avoided.

Tips for Dining Out

1) To avoid overeating, have a light snack before going to a restaurant. Grab something light, like vegetables or turkey roll ups.
2) If you can't resist complimentary bread baskets or bowls of tortilla chips, you can politely ask your server to remove them. If your order of salsa, hummus or guacamole comes with chips or bread, ask if you can substitute sliced veggies instead.
3) Avoid high-carb options like fries, pasta salad or other high-carb sides. Ask for low-carb substitutes like asparagus or broccoli.
4) Avoid salads that come in shells (like tortilla) and go easy on the add-ons. Make sure that any meat in your salad is grilled, not breaded or fried. If you are in Phase 1, also avoid particularly high-carb fruits like grapes and mango.
5) Sandwich bread is a source of unnecessary carbohydrates; ask if your sandwich can be made into a salad or lettuce wrap. If not, limit yourself to the sandwich filling, or remove one slice for an open-faced option if you are in the later phases of Atkins.

Snack Choices

Try to keep your snacks healthy by making snacks out of any/all the foods previously listed in the chapter. Choose foods for your snack based on the phase of the Atkins diet that you are currently following. Also try to follow a routine or set number of snacks per day, for example 2 snacks a day. Make sure not to over-snack as that may be detrimental to your routine. Pack snacks in small containers or zip-top bags so you can track your intake of Net Carbohydrates. Here are some snacking options:

- Veggies with salad dressing
- Ham or turkey rollups
- Greek yogurt with berries
- Nuts, Olives
- Smoked salmon rolls
- Cheese, Hard-boiled eggs
- Atkins bars and shakes

Chapter 4 Using a Slow Cooker on Atkins Diet

What is Slow Cooking?
Slow cooking is a very old food preparation technique; it simply refers to cooking food on low temperatures for a longer period. This method yields tender meats, thick sauces and a depth of flavor that can be hard to achieve with other techniques. Recipes for slow-cooking are often referred to as 'one-pot 'recipes because all the ingredients involved are just cut into pieces and put into the cooking vessel. Add some liquid and seasoning, and it's ready to go. Once you turn the cooker on, there is no need to stir or check on the food.

Benefits of Slow Cooking
Nutritious Meals: The slow cooking method results in scrumptious meals made from fresh ingredients. When cooked at low temperatures, your food won't dry out, so you will end up with juicy vegetables or a very tender cut of meat.

Saving Time: You don't have stand over your slow cooker or check on it. Just put the ingredients in and turn the cooker on; now you can work on other things while your food cooks. This is why working parents adopt slow-cooking for everyday meals.

Low Heat: Your slow cooker generates very little external heat compared to an oven or stovetop, making it an ideal choice for cooking during hot weather.

Energy Efficiency: Slow-cookers consume much less energy compared to conventional ovens or stovetops. They can even operate on solar panel energy!

Easy Cleanup: After the prep for your slow-cooker meal, the only things to clean are a cutting board, a couple knives and the stoneware slow-cooker insert; no more piles of pots and pans.

FAQs of Slow Cooking

Q: Is slow-cooking a safe cooking technique?

A: Slow-cookers normally heat up to 209°F; that, along with the moisture in the pot over the long cooking time, kills common bacteria, so your meal will be safe.

Q: What is the difference between the High and Low temperature settings?

A: The difference is the time it takes for the slow cooker to heat up to 209°F. On the High setting, it's 4 hours, and on the Low setting it's 8 hours. After that, the cooking time depends on the size and weight of the pieces to be cooked.

Q: What is the normal cooking time for a slow-cooker?

A: On the High setting, most dishes will take 3 to 4 hours. On the Low setting, most dishes take 7 to 8 hours. However, this will vary significantly depending on the recipe you're following.

Q: How long should a whole chicken take to cook?

A: In general, a 6-pound chicken takes 7.5 hours on Low and 6 hours on High.

Q: Does the food need to be stirred while cooking?

A: In general, no stirring is needed, which is a major advantage of slow-cooking. However, always double-check your specific recipe as some dishes will vary.

Q: Can I open the lid while food is cooking?

A: It is not recommended to remove the slow-cooker lid while your food is cooking; the slow cooker will lose heat, and your dish will take longer to cook.

Q: Is it safe to leave the slow-cooker on, unattended?

A: Yes, it is safe to leave the slow-cooker on, but it is recommended to use the Low setting in this case.

Q: Can the stoneware pot used on the stove top?

A: No, the stoneware cannot withstand direct heat and will crack. However, it is safe to be used in the microwave.

Q: What size of pot should I buy?

A: That depends on the number of people you're feeding, and the size of the meat cuts you may wish to prepare. Visit a store and check the physical size of the different slow cookers so you know what will fit.

30 Easy-to-Follow Slow Cooker Recipes for the Atkins Diet

Following a strict Atkins diet can be difficult if you are used to eating out or ordering delivery. You'll need to take charge and learn to make some delicious recipes for yourself. But don't worry, we've got you covered! Here are some easy and delicious recipes.

1. Simple and Delicious Chicken Enchiladas

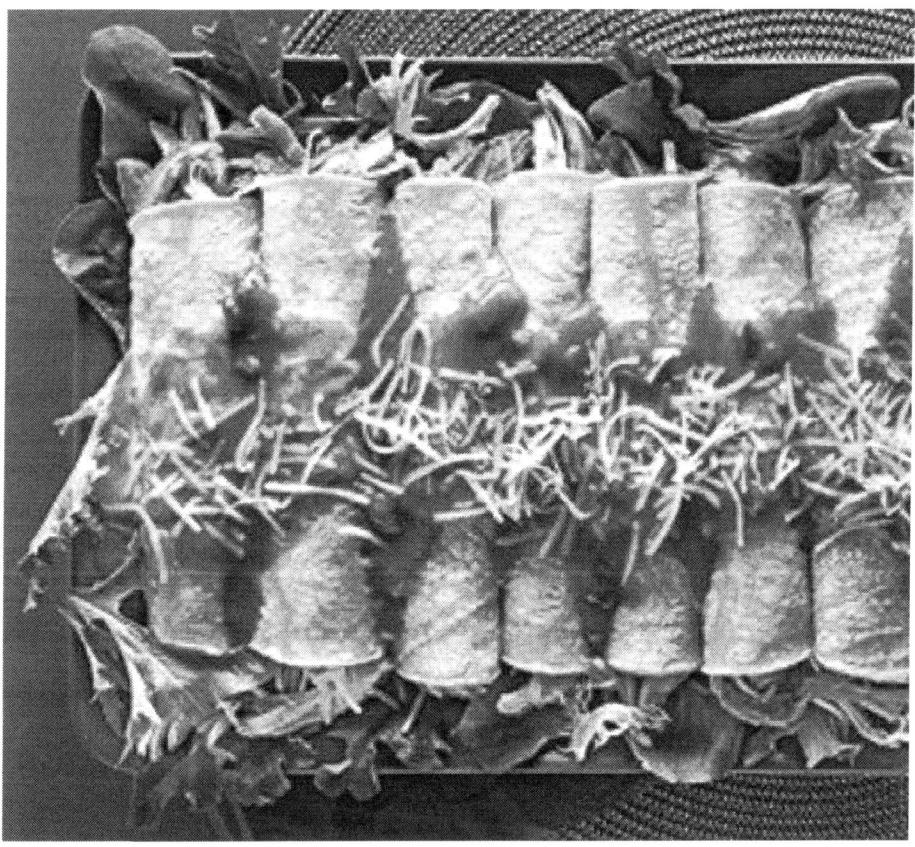

Ingredients

- 10 ½ oz. Cream of Chicken soup (reduced fat)
- 1 lb. boneless chicken breasts, skinless and cut in half
- 1/2 cup salsa
- diced green chilies to taste (they're hot!)
- 1 teaspoon chili powder
- 1/2 teaspoon ground cumin
- 4 cups packaged baby lettuce mix

- 2-4 warmed corn tortillas (warm in the microwave and wrap in a towel until serving)
- 1/2 cup shredded cheese blend

Instructions

1. Place chicken in the slow cooker.
2. In a small bowl, combine the soup, salsa, chilies and cumin. Mix well and pour the mixture over the chicken.
3. Cover the cooker and cook on the Low setting for 4- 5 hours.
4. Remove the chicken breasts and shred with two forks. Add some of the sauce from the cooker until you have a saucy enchilada filling.
5. Cover a large serving plate with the lettuce mix. Place a few spoonfuls of chicken mixture into the centre of a tortilla; top with lettuce, roll up and place on the platter. Repeat with remaining tortillas. Spoon the remaining sauce over the enchiladas and sprinkle cheese on top. Serve.

Nutrition Value: Protein: 36.2 g, Fat: 19.8 g, Carbohydrate: 3.4 g, Fiber: 5.0g **Total Calories:** 351.3

2. Easy Heart-Warming Caramel Rolls

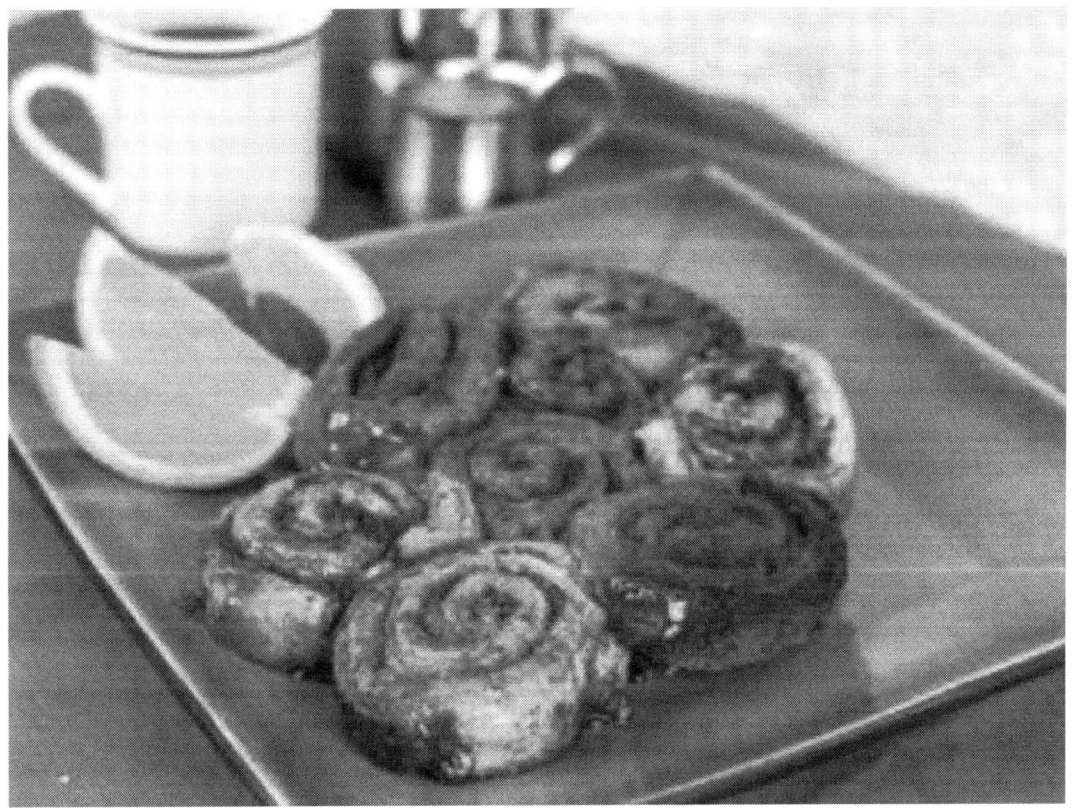

Ingredients

- 1 package refrigerated cinnamon rolls
- 4 Tbsp. butter
- 1/2 cup brown sugar

Instructions

1. Spray the inside of the stoneware insert with cooking spray.

2. In a small saucepan over low-to-medium heat, melt the butter. Add the brown sugar. Let cook, stirring the caramel sauce occasionally, until it's thick and smooth - about 3 minutes.

3. Open the package of cinnamon rolls, separate and form the rolls according to manufacturer instructions. Place the rolls into the bottom of the slow cooker and pour the caramel sauce over them. Cover and cook for an hour on High. Enjoy these warm and tender caramel rolls.

Nutrition Value: Protein: 2g, Fat: 15g, Carbohydrate: 6g, Fiber: 0g
Total Calories: 245

3. Unforgettable Slow-Cooker Tater Tots

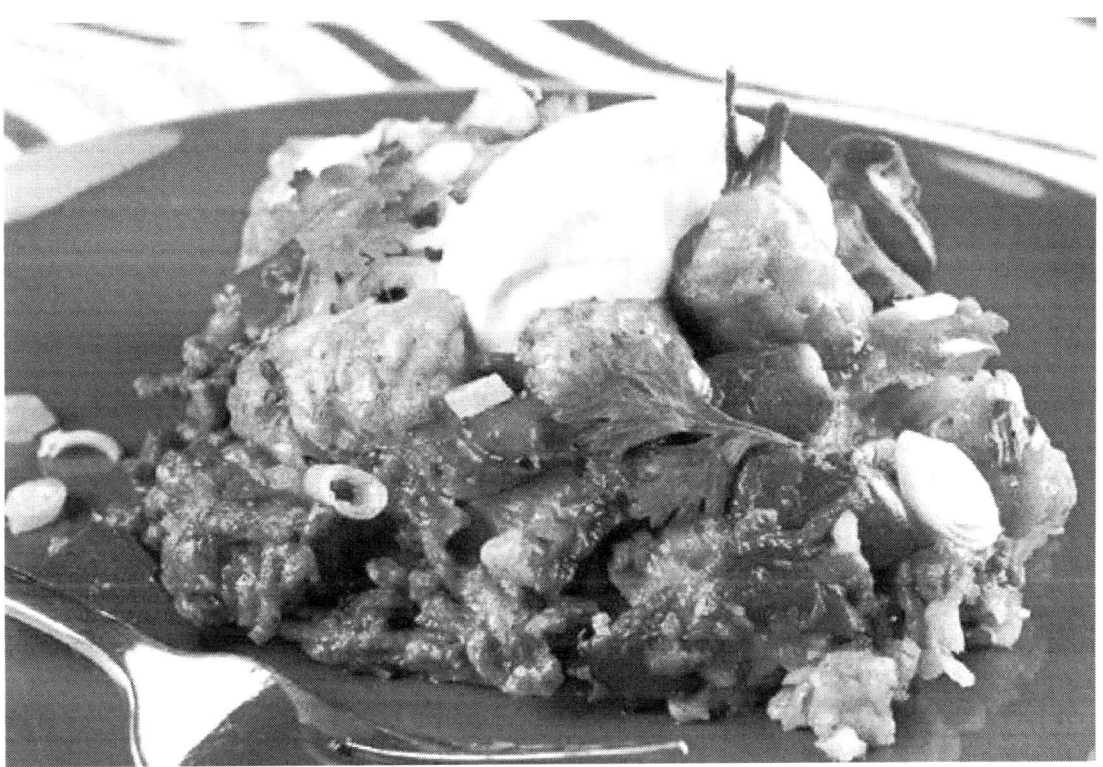

Ingredients

- 15 oz. Tater Tots
- 3 oz. Canadian bacon, diced
- 1 onion, chopped
- ½ cup cheddar cheese, shredded
- 1/8 cup Parmesan cheese, grated
- 6 eggs
- ½ cup milk
- 2 Tbsp. all-purpose flour
- ½ tsp. salt
- 1/4 tsp. pepper

Instructions

1. Grease the stoneware insert with butter or ghee and add, one at a time in layers, 1/3 of the Tots, onion, bacon and cheeses. Repeat with the two remaining thirds.
2. In a large bowl, mix together all the remaining ingredients. Pour the mixture over the layered ingredients.
3. Cover and cook on Low for 6-8 hours.

You can prepare this overnight and enjoy a ready-made breakfast in the morning!

Nutrition Value: Protein: 40.9g, Fat: 37.6g, Carbohydrate: 12g, Fiber: 38.3g **Total Calories:** 654

4. Delicious Sausage and Egg Casserole

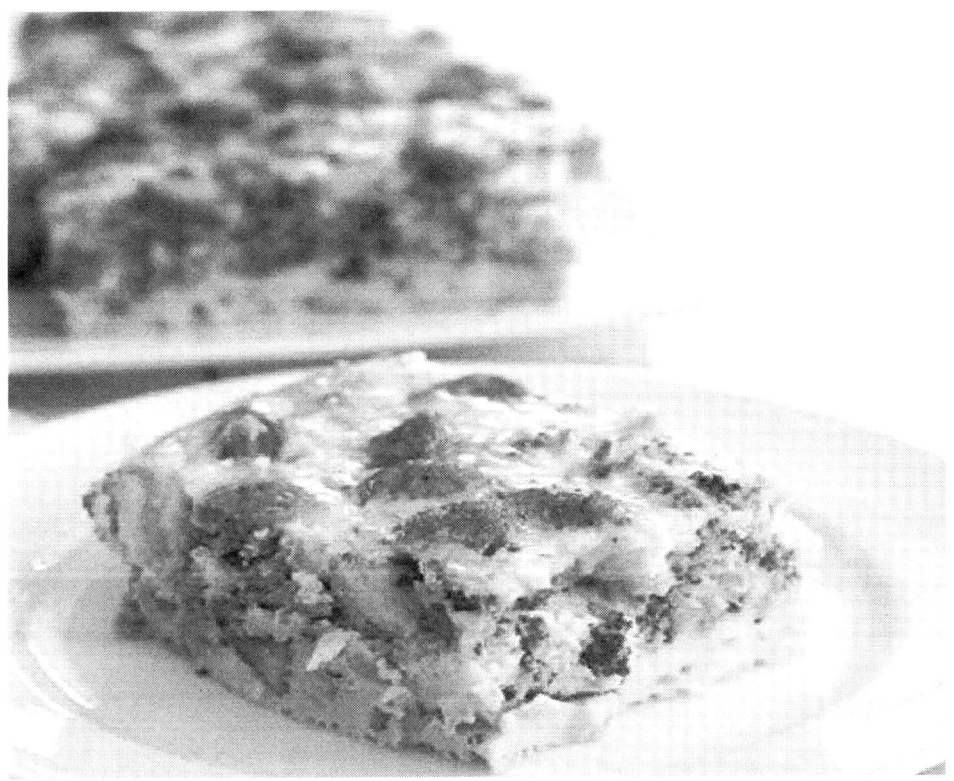

Ingredients

- 1 medium head broccoli, chopped
- 12 oz. low-carb sausages, cooked and sliced
- 1 cup shredded Cheddar cheese, divided
- 10 Eggs
- 2 cloves garlic, minced
- 1/2 tsp salt
- 1/4 tsp pepper
- 3/4 cup whipping cream

Instructions:

1) Grease the inside of the stoneware insert.
2) Add, one at a time in layers, ½ of the broccoli, sausage and cheese. Repeat with the remaining ingredients.
3) In a large bowl, add the garlic, whipping cream, eggs, salt and pepper and whisk them together until well combined. Pour the egg mixture over the layered ingredients.
4) Cover and cook on High for 2-3 hours. The casserole is ready when the edges are browned, and it is set in the center. Enjoy!

Nutrition Value: Protein: 13.2 g, Fat: 15.4 g, Carbohydrate: 7.6 g, Fiber: 0.6 g **Total Calories:** 223.6

5. Tempting Breakfast Casserole with Tomato and Spinach

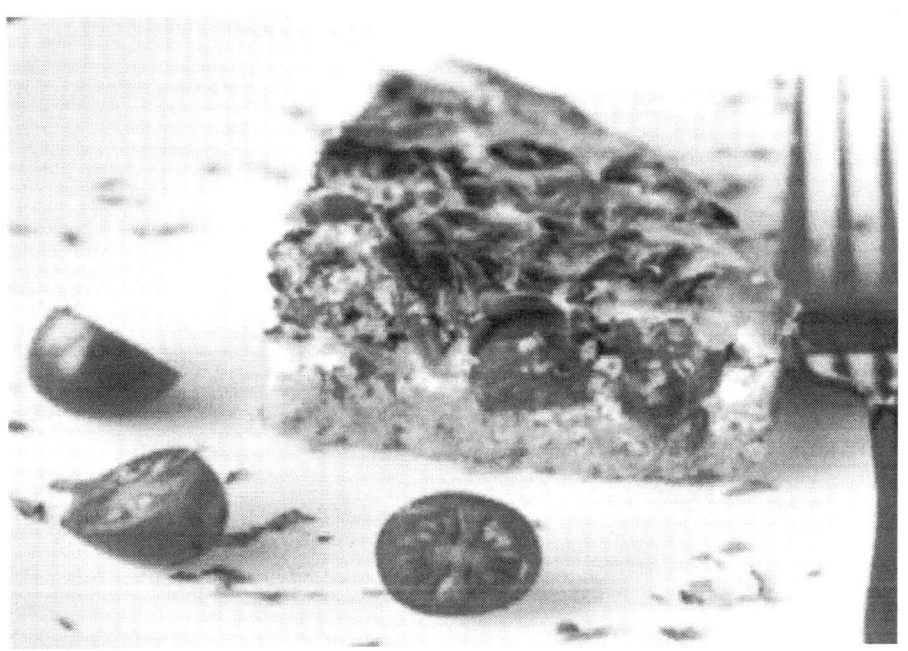

Ingredients

- ¼ cup uncooked quinoa
- ½ cup milk
- 3 large eggs
- Salt and pepper to taste
- Handful of fresh spinach
- ½ cup of tomatoes
- 1/8 cup shredded cheese of your choice
- 1/8 cup Parmesan cheese

Instructions
1. In a mixing bowl, add the quinoa, milk, salt and pepper and eggs and stir until combined.
2. Add the spinach, tomatoes and half of the cheese and stir to combine.

3. Grease the stoneware insert and pour in the mixture
4. Sprinkle the Parmesan cheese over the top.
5. Cover and cook for 3-4 hours until the edges are browned, and the eggs are set in the center.

Nutrition Value: Protein: 16.2 g, Fat: 9.3 g, Carbohydrate: 2.2 g, Fiber: 3.7 g **Total Calories:** 188.2

6. Scrumptious Breakfast Pie

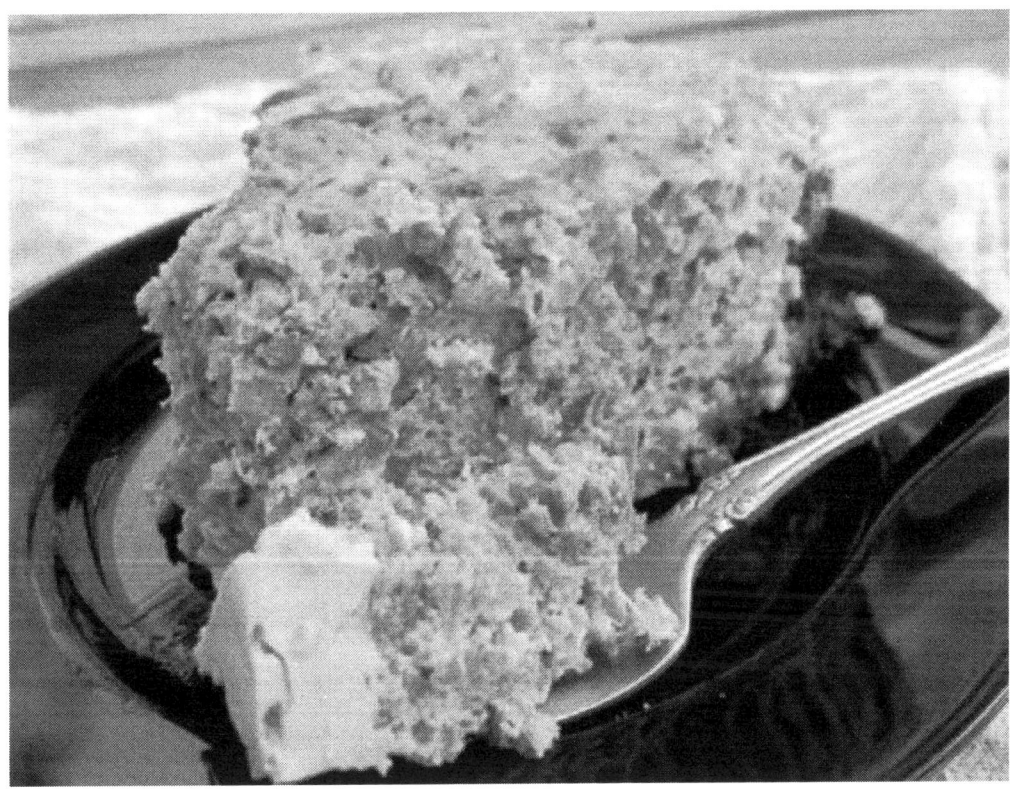

Ingredients

- 4 eggs
- 1 small sweet potato, shredded
- ½ lb. pork breakfast sausage, broken up
- 1 small yellow onion, diced
- ½ Tbsp. garlic powder
- 1 tsp dried basil
- salt and pepper, to taste
- Chopped bell peppers or any other green veggie you want to add.

Instructions

1. Grease the stoneware insert.
2. Shred the sweet potato with a box grater and place in the slow cooker.
3. Add the rest of the ingredients and stir well.
4. Cook on Low for 6-7 hours. Make sure that the pork sausages are thoroughly cooked. Enjoy!

Nutrition Value: Protein: 7.8 g, Fat: 10.8 g, Carbohydrate: 2.8 g, Fiber: 4.1 g **Total Calories:** 234.2

7. Tender Autumn Oxtail Stew

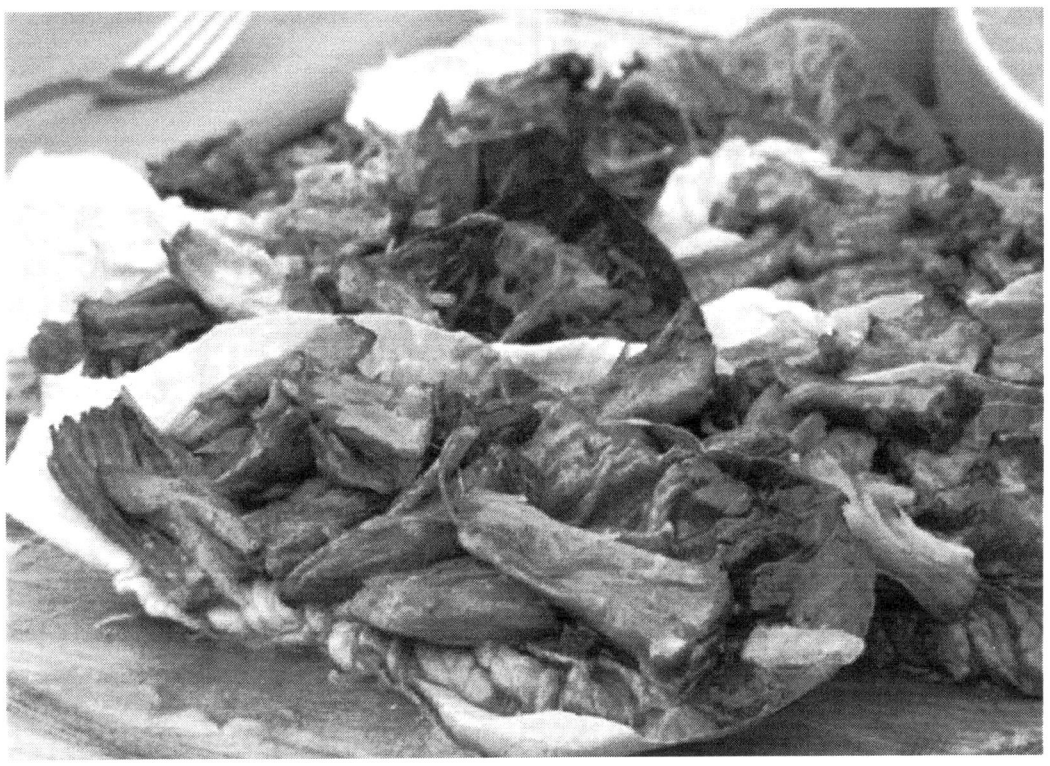

Ingredients

- 1 kg (2.2 lbs.) oxtail or stewing beef
- 1 Tbsp. butter or lard
- 1 cup beef stock or water
- 1 small red onion
- 1 garlic head
- 1 carrot
- 1 celery stalk
- A splash of fresh orange juice and some peel
- 1 cinnamon stick
- A pinch of nutmeg

- 5 cloves
- 1 dried or fresh bay leaf
- black pepper and salt to taste
- 2 heads small lettuce

Instructions

1. Season the oxtail or beef with salt and pepper, place on a baking sheet and bake at 150 C / 300 F for 30 mins, until browned. Alternatively, you can brown the oxtail on the stove, in a frying pan.
2. Peel the carrot, onion and garlic. Mince the garlic and roughly chop the carrot and onion.
3. In a small pot, add the beef stock, orange juice and spices; bring to a boil, simmer for 5 minutes, remove from heat and set aside.
4. Place the browned oxtail in the slow cooker; add the rest of the ingredients and cook on Low for 3-4. The oxtail is done when it's fork-tender.
5. Turn off the slow cooker and remove the oxtail, discarding all the spices and the vegetables (or save them to use in another dish)
6. Shred the meat with two forks and serve on a bed of lettuce. Enjoy!

Nutrition value: Net Carbohydrates 4g, fiber 1.4g, protein 54.4g, fat 49.5g **Total Calories:** 693

8. Delicious Slow Cooked Poached Salmon

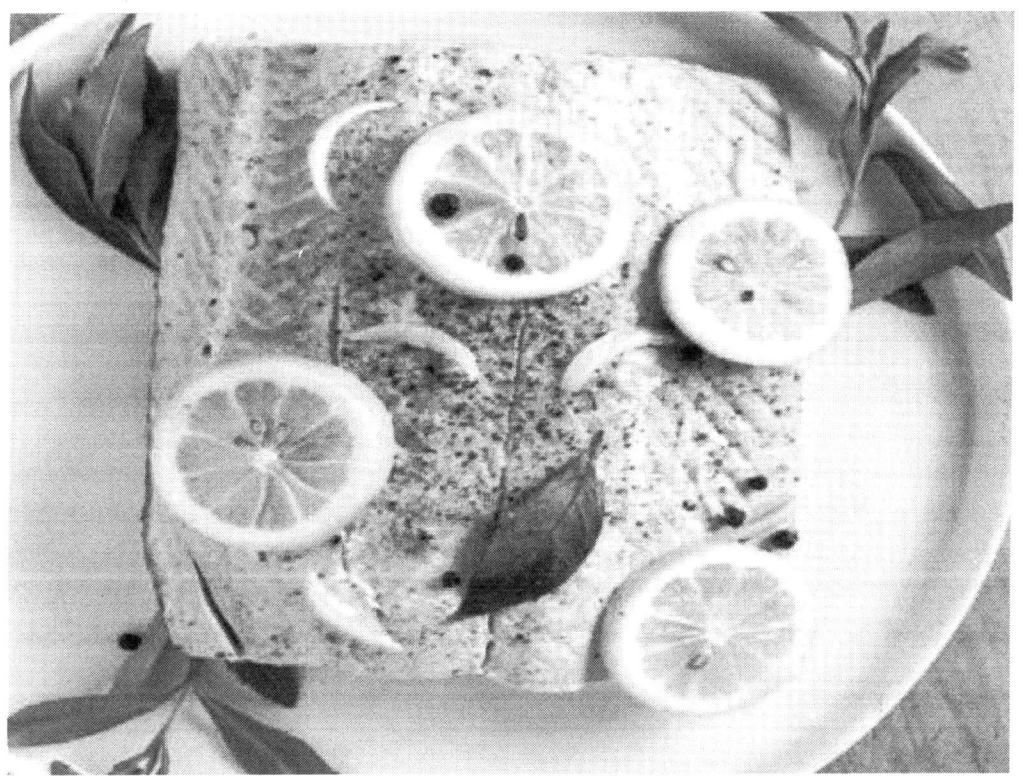

Ingredients

- 1 cup water
- ½ cup dry white wine
- 1 shallot, thinly sliced
- Any fresh herb of your choice
- ½ tsp black peppercorns
- 1 lemon, thinly sliced
- ½ tsp kosher salt
- 1 pounds salmon, skin on
- olive oil for serving

Instructions:

1. In a small pot, add the water, bay leaf, herbs, lemon, shallots, wine, peppercorns. Bring to a boil and simmer 30 mins.
2. Season the salmon on both sides with salt & pepper to taste.
3. Place the salmon in the slow cooker, skin side. Cover and cook on High for 30-45 min. Check if the salmon is cooked to your preference.
4. Once done, take out the salmon and lightly drizzle with olive oil. Garnish with lemon slices and serve.

Nutrition value: Fat: 30.5 g, Carbohydrates: 1.5 g, Fiber: 0.2 g, Protein: 46.5 g **Total Calories:** 504

9. Delicious Slow-cooked Italian Beef

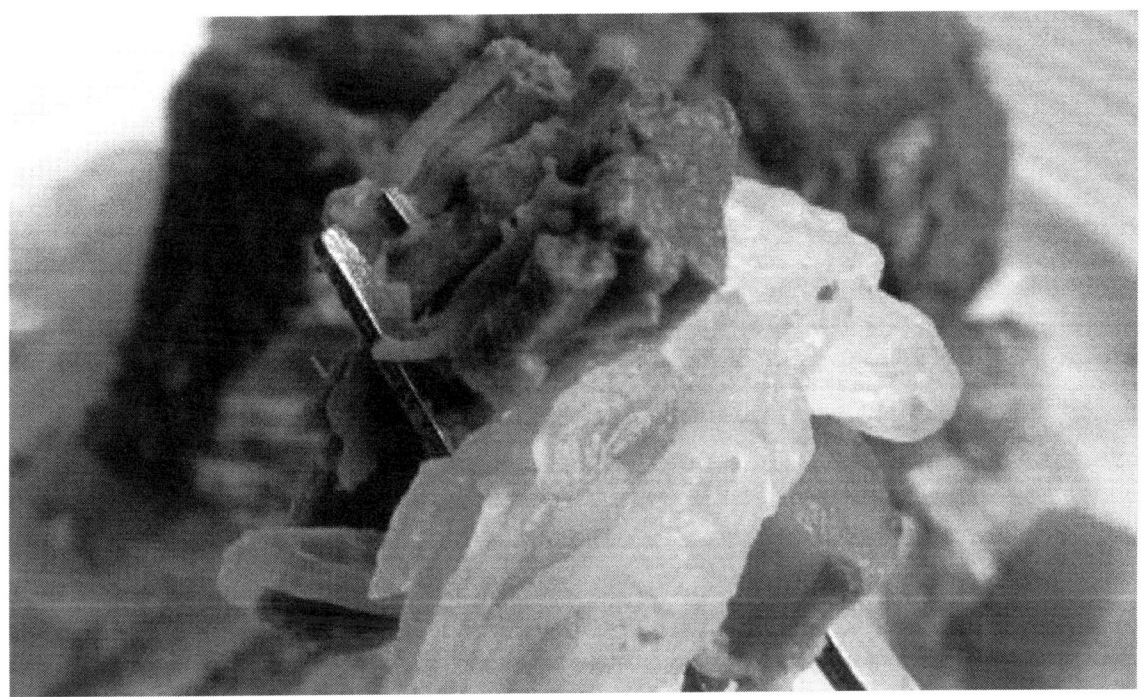

Ingredients

- 2 lbs. beef roast
- ½ cup chopped carrots
- 1 small white or yellow onion, sliced
- 3-4 cloves garlic, chopped
- ½ tsp kosher salt
- ½ tsp garlic powder
- ½ tsp dried basil
- ½ tsp dried oregano
- ¼ tsp dried thyme
- Pinch of ground cinnamon
- Pinch of red chili flakes
- 1 cup organic crushed tomatoes
- 1 cup beef stock

- 1 cup tomato paste

Instructions

1. Cut the beef into 1" pieces, trimming any extra fat, and place in the slow cooker.
2. Wash, peel and slice the vegetables; add all remaining ingredients to the slow cooker. Stir to dissolve the tomato paste into the beef stock.
3. Cover and cook on High for 5-6 hours or until the beef is fork-tender.
4. Serve with a side of roasted vegetables or legumes.

Nutrition value: Net Carbohydrates 1.2 g, fiber 0g, protein 32.4 g, fat 5.9 g **Total Calories:** 197.0

10. Mouthwatering Chicken and Kale Soup

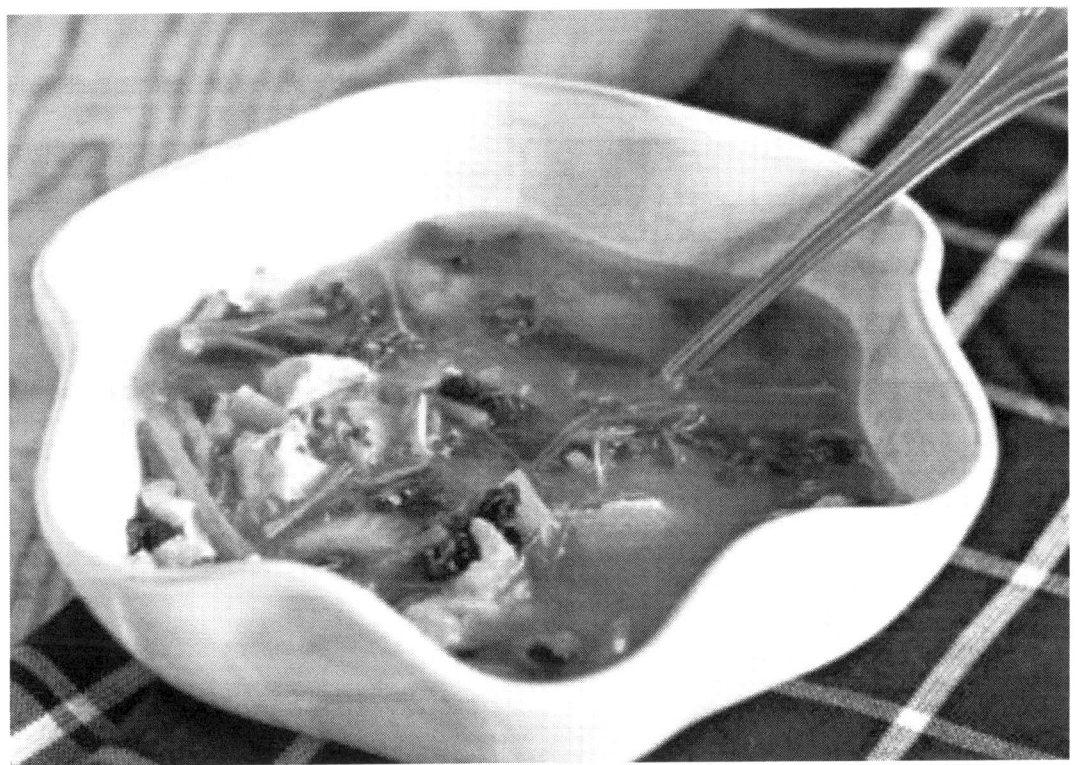

Ingredients:

- 6 boneless skinless chicken thighs or breasts
- 3 1/2 cups of chicken broth
- 1/2 large onion, chopped
- 4 smashed cloves of garlic
- 1 1/2 cups carrots, shredded
- 4 cups of chopped kale
- 1 1/2 tsp fresh or dried parsley
- salt and pepper to taste

Instructions:

1. Place the chicken, onion, garlic and chicken broth in the slow cooker.
2. Cover and cook on Low for 4 to 6 hours, until the chicken is tender and falling apart. Add the rest of the ingredients, shred the chicken with two forks, cover and let cook for another hour.
3. Enjoy your hearty meal!

Nutrition Value: Protein: 7 g, Fat: 12 g, Carbohydrate: 7 g, Fiber: 1 g **Total Calories:** 69

11. Appetizing Orange Chicken

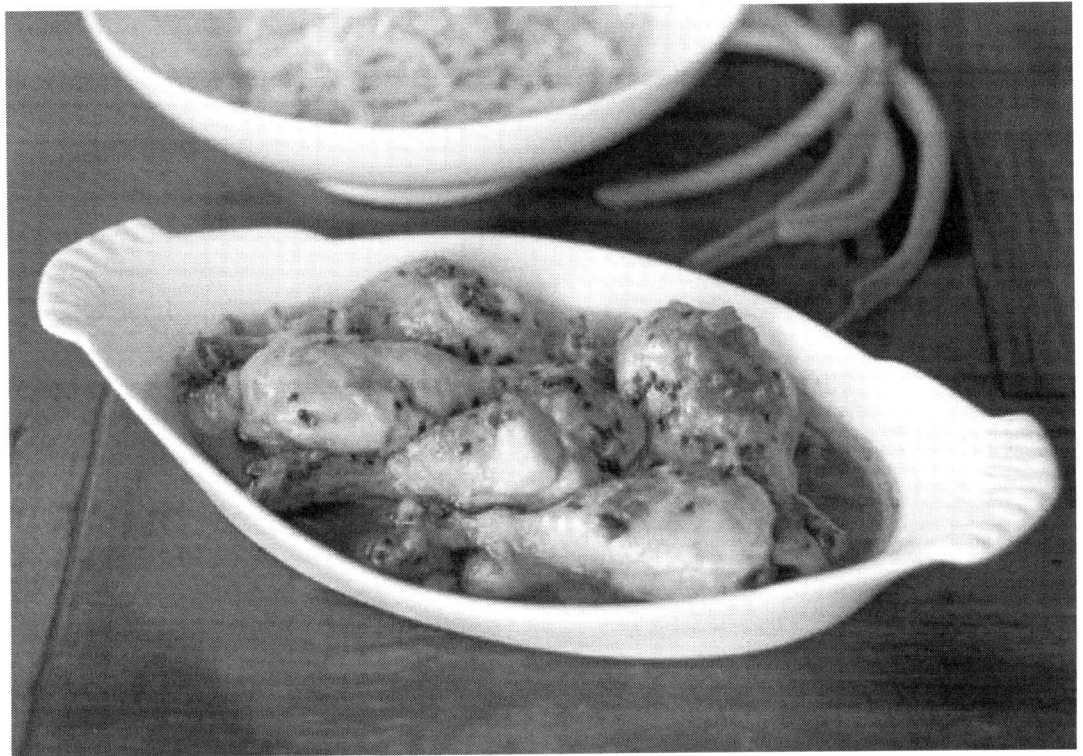

Ingredients

- ¼ cup melted butter or coconut oil
- ¼ cup coconut milk
- 2 Tbsp. Swerve Confectioners
- 1 tsp sesame oil (toasted)
- 1 tsp organic soy sauce
- ½ tsp fresh ginger, grated
- ½ tsp sesame seeds
- ½ tsp orange extract
- ¼ tsp fish sauce
- 1½ ls bone-in chicken thighs or breasts
- 1 Tbsp. black sesame seeds (optional)

- 4 spring onions, sliced

Instructions:

1. In a small bowl, combine all ingredients (other than the chicken) and whisk until smooth.
2. Cook the chicken in the slow cooker for 4-5 hours on Low until it is soft but not falling apart.
3. Pour over the sauce, cover and cook for another 30 mins to 1 hour.
4. Garnish with back sesame and spring onions.

Nutrition Value: Protein: 34g, Fat: 32g, Carbohydrate: 1.1g, Fiber: 0 g
Total Calories: 491

12. Delightful Garlic Butter Chicken with Cream Cheese Sauce

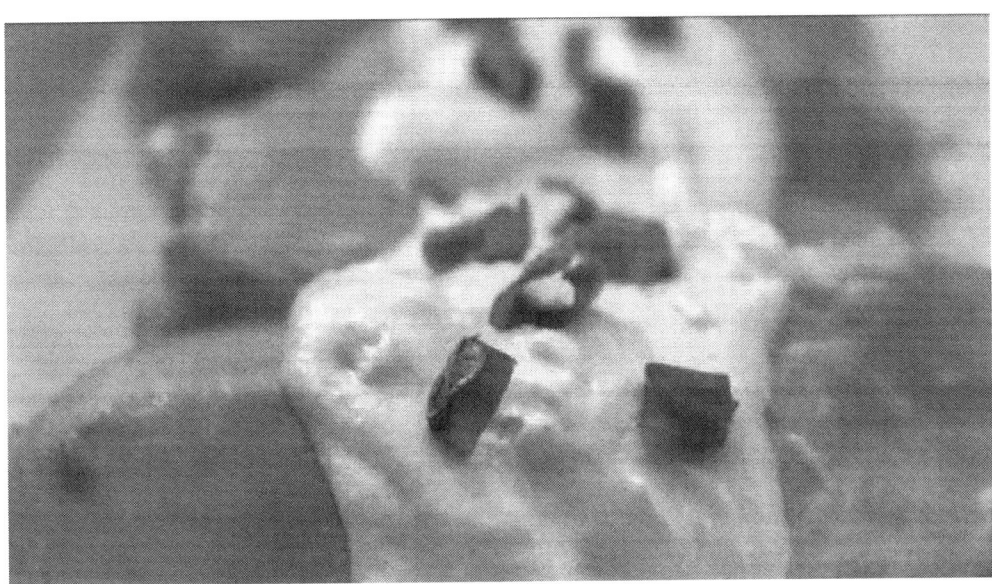

Ingredients

- 2 lbs. boneless chicken breasts or thighs
- ½ stick of butter
- 4 garlic cloves, sliced
- 1 tsp salt or to taste
- 1 small onion, sliced
- 4 oz. cream cheese
- ½ cup chicken stock. (You can also use the liquid left in the slow cooker after the chicken is cooked)
- salt to taste

Instructions

For the garlic chicken:

1. Place the chicken in the slow cooker.
2. Add in the butter, garlic and salt, distributing evenly in the cooker.
3. Cover and cook on Low for 6 hours.

4. Once the chicken is done, take it out and place it on a serving dish.

For the cream cheese sauce:

1. Put the chicken stock or the liquid from the cooker into a medium saucepan.
2. Add in the cream cheese and salt.
3. Cook on medium heat until the sauce is creamy and well combined. Serve hot with the chicken.

Nutrition Value: Protein: 28.2 g, Fat: 21.3 g, Carbohydrate: 7.9 g, Fiber: 1.1 g **Total Calories:** 169.3

13. Slow-cooked Brats

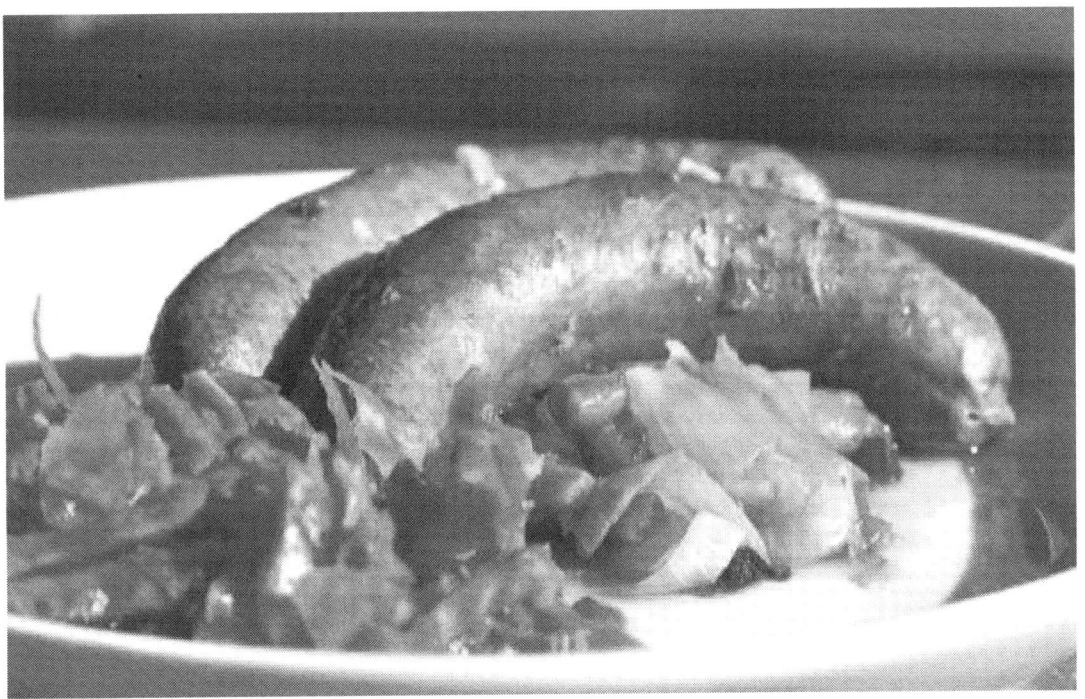

Ingredients

- 1 package of Bison Brats
- 1 medium onion, sliced
- 1 cup bell pepper, cut into strips
- 1 cup homemade chicken or beef broth
- Dried herbs of your choice, such as thyme, basil, parsley
- Any hot sauce, to taste
- Salt to taste

Instructions

1. Place the sliced onions and peppers in the bottom of the slow cooker.

2. Layer the brats overtop.
3. Add the broth , spices and hot sauce.
4. Cover and cook on Low for 4-6 hours, or on High for 30 minutes
5. Serve with organic cooked rice

Nutrition Value: Protein: 26 g, Fat: 50 g, Carbohydrate: 5 g, Fiber: 2 g
Total Calories: 733

14. Creamy Reuben Soup

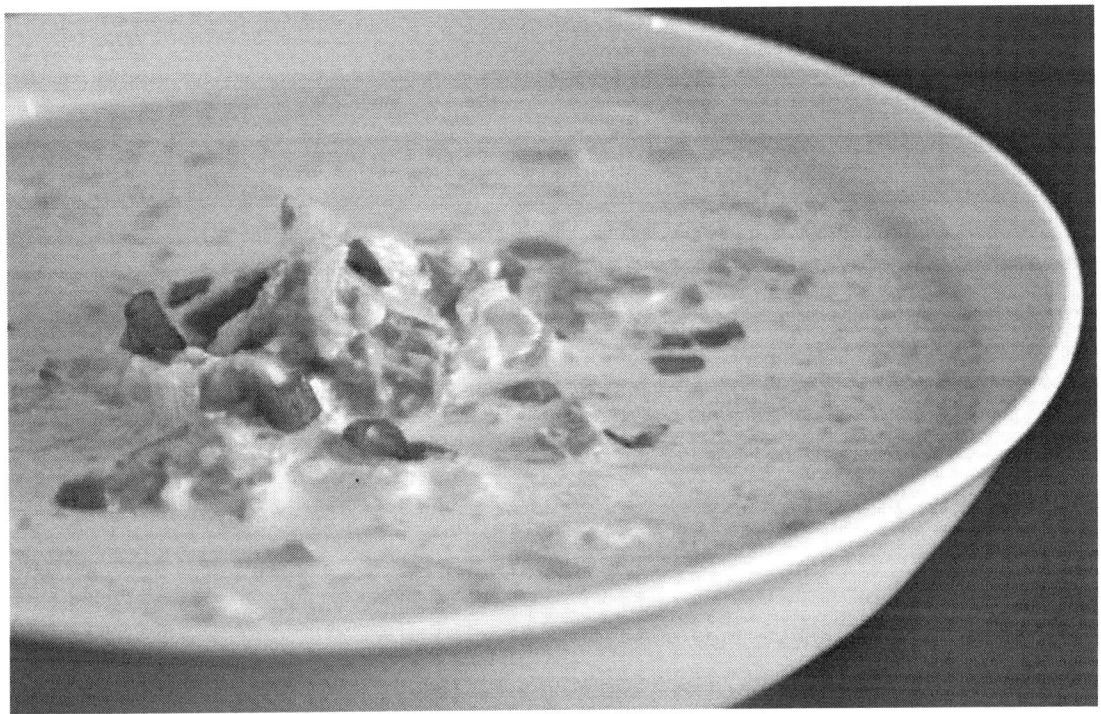

Ingredients

- 1 small onion, diced
- 1 rib celery, diced
- 1 large cloves garlic, minced
- 1 ½ Tbsp. butter
- 1/2 lb. corned beef, chopped
- 2 cups homemade or 'clean' beef stock
- ½ cup sauerkraut
- ½ tsp sea salt
- ½ tsp caraway seeds
- ½ tsp black pepper
- 1 cup heavy cream
- 1 ½ cups Swiss cheese, shredded

Instructions

1. Start heating the slow cooker on High.
2. In a large sauté pan, add onions, celery, butter and garlic and cook over low-medium heat until soft and translucent. Transfer to slow cooker.
3. Add corned beef, sauerkraut, sea salt, beef stock, caraway seed and black pepper to the slow cooker.
4. Cover and cook on High for 4-5 hours.
5. When the beef is almost done, add heavy cream and Swiss cheese and cook 1 additional hour.

Nutrition Value: Protein: 11.5g, Fat: 18.5g, Carbohydrate: 4g, Fiber: 0 g **Total Calories:** 225

15. Tasty Slow-cooked Pesto Chicken Salad

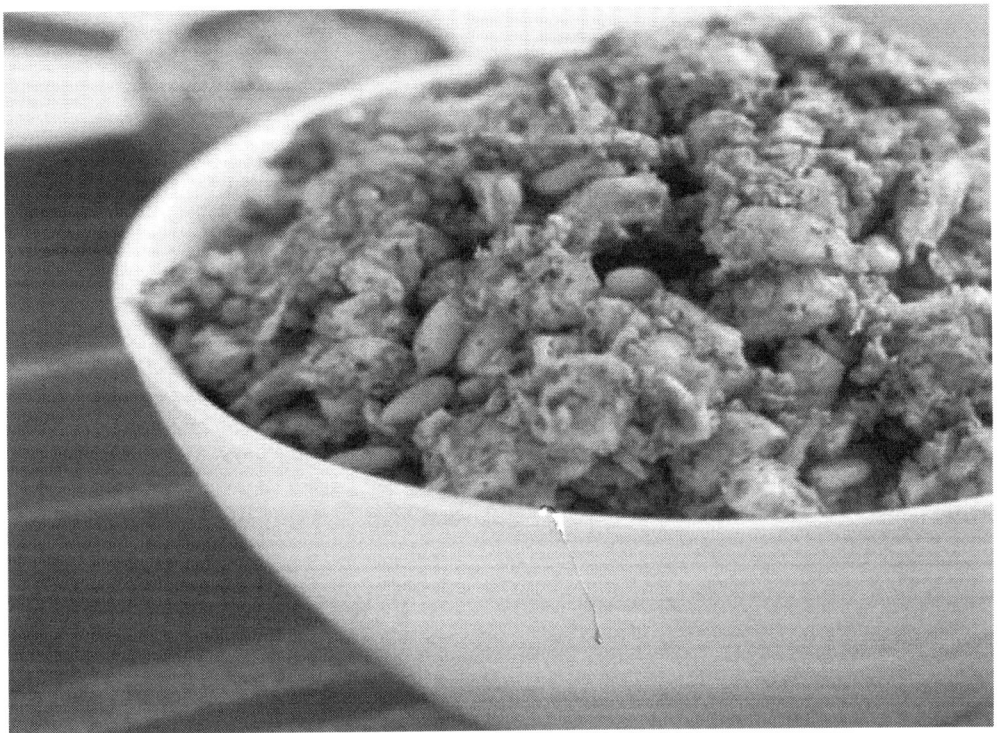

Ingredients

- 3 or 4 chicken breasts
- 1 garlic clove, chopped
- 1 small sized white onion, chopped
- 1 cup organic preferably homemade chicken broth
- 1/4 teaspoon garlic powder
- Pinch of salt and ground pepper to taste
- ¼ cup pine nuts for garnishing
- 1/2 cup cashews, walnuts, or nuts of choice
- 1 cup basil
- 1 1/2 cup spinach
- 1 Tbsp. virgin olive oil
- 1 garlic clove

- 1/2 lemon, juiced
- Salt and pepper to taste

Instructions

1. Place the chicken, garlic, onion, broth and seasoning into the slow cooker and cook on High for 4-5 hours.
2. Meanwhile, prepare the pesto sauce. Place the nuts, basil, spinach, olive oil, garlic clove, lemon juice, salt and pepper in a food processor and process until smooth.
3. Shred the chicken with two forks; place in a bowl, add the pesto sauce and stir to combine.
4. In a small pan, toast the pine nuts for 3-4 minutes, constantly stirring to avoid burning.
5. Garnish the pesto chicken salad with the pine nuts and serve.

Nutrition Value: Protein: 10.1 g, Fat: 6.9 g, Carbohydrate: 1.4 g, Fiber: 1.7 g **Total Calories:** 144.4

16. Delicious Stuffed Poblano Peppers

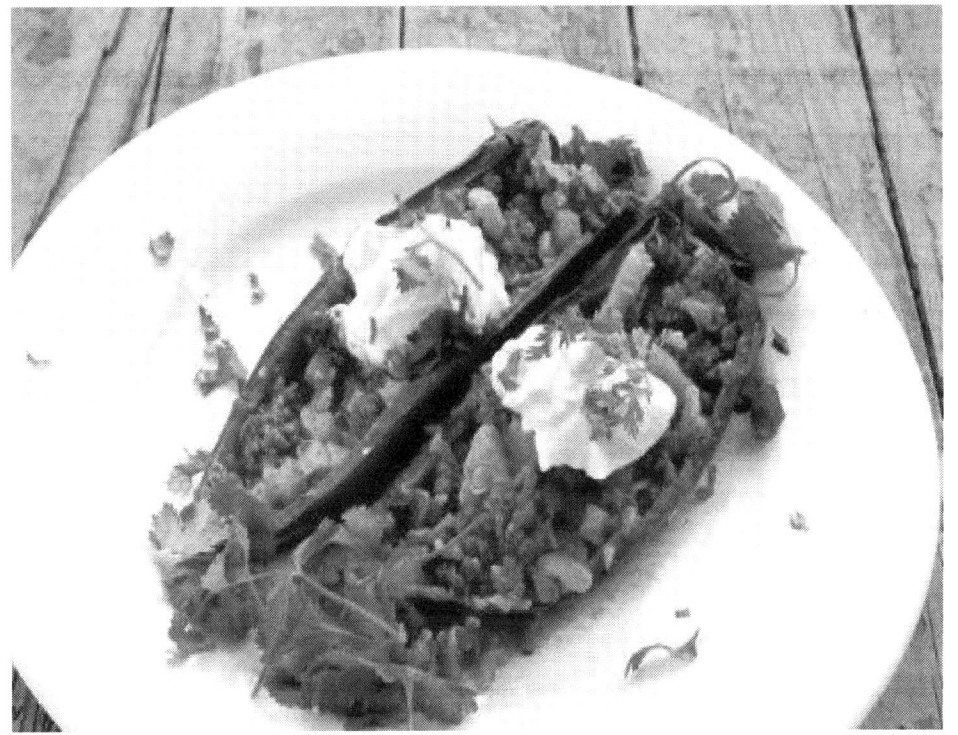

Ingredients

- 1 poblano pepper
- 1 Tbsp. chopped onion
- 1 cup tomato juice
- 3 Tbsp. tomato sauce
- 1/3 cup finely chopped cauliflower
- 1/3 lb. ground beef

Instructions
1. In a medium bowl, combine the beef, onion, cauliflower and tomato sauce.
2. Place 1/2 inch of tomato juice in the slow cooker.

3. Stuff the peppers with the beef mixture and carefully place the stuffed peppers into the cooker.
4. Cook on Low for about 4 hours or until the meat is cooked and tender.

Nutrition Value: Protein: 21.7 g, Fat: 13.7 g, Carbohydrate: 6.8 g, Fiber: 5.2 g **Total Calories:** 314.6

17. Yummy Cheesy Roasted Brussels dip

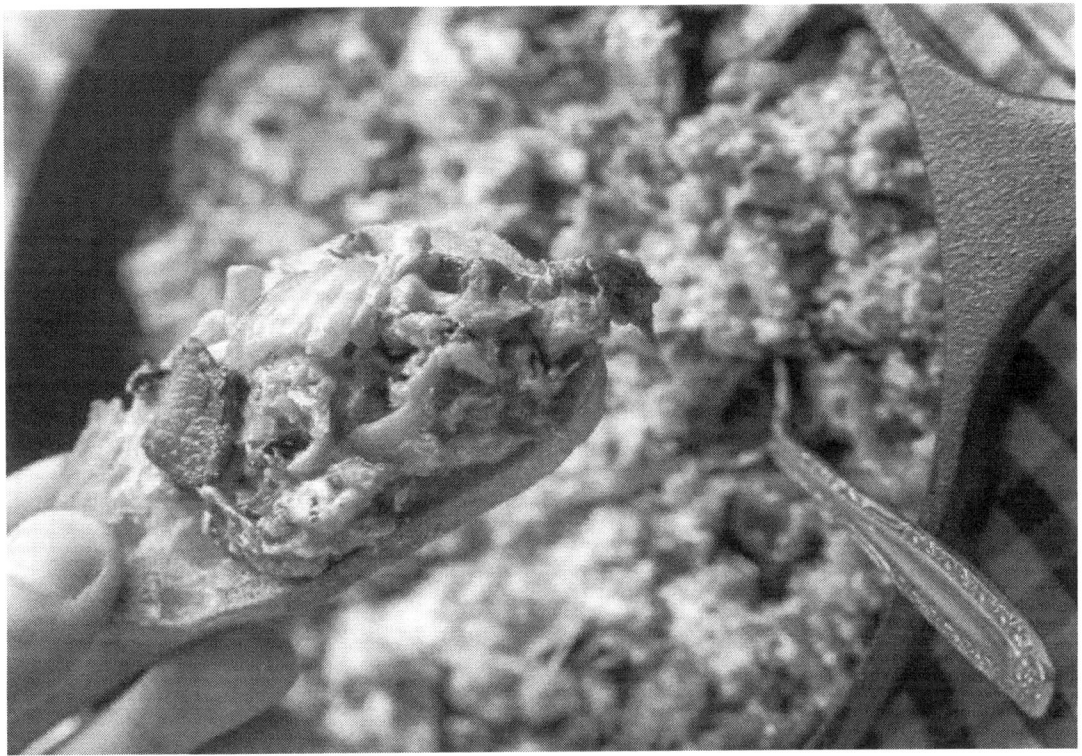

Ingredients

- ½ lb. Brussels sprouts, chopped
- ½ Tbsp. olive oil
- 1 clove of peeled and crushed garlic
- ¼ tsp fresh thyme, chopped
- 2 ounces cream cheese
- 1/8 cup sour cream
- 1/8 cup mayonnaise
- ½ cup mozzarella cheese, shredded
- 1/8 cup parmesan cheese, grated
- salt and pepper to taste

Instructions

1. Literally toss all the ingredients into the cooker (trust us!).
2. Cover the cooker and cook for 1-2 hours on Low. It's done when the cheese is nice and melted.

Nutrition Value: Protein: 13 g, Fat: 33g, Carbohydrate: 12g, Fiber: 4 g
Total Calories: 396

18. Heavenly Braised Cabbage

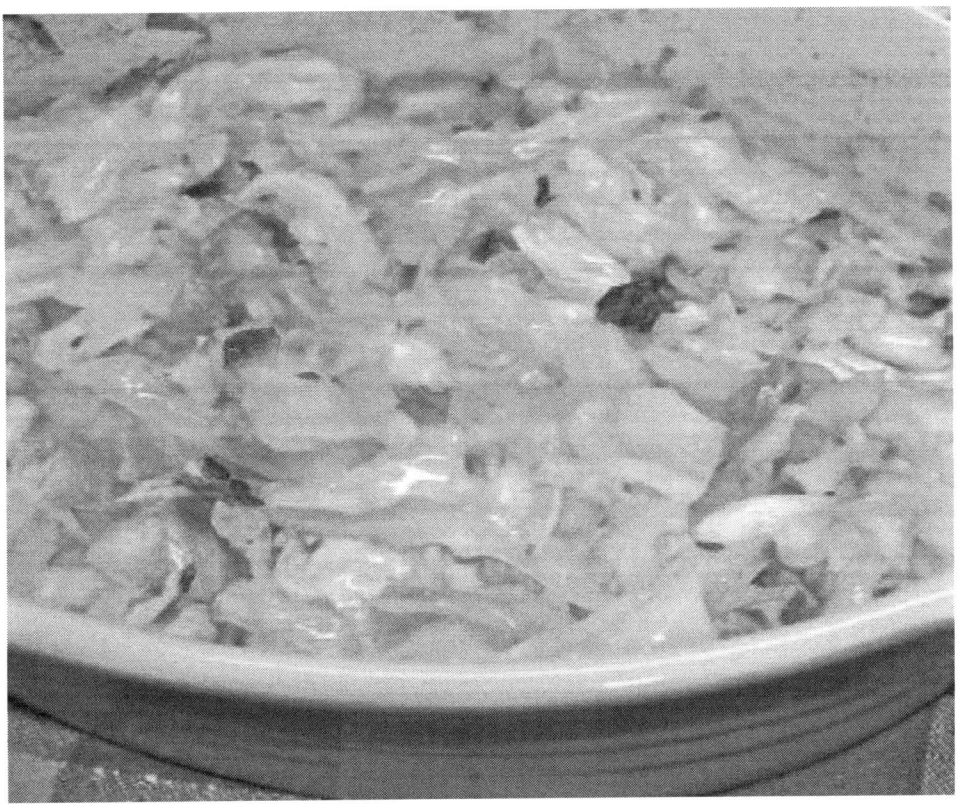

Ingredients

- 1 head green cabbage
- 1 large sweet onion, sliced
- ¼-½ cup bone broth
- Sea salt to taste
- ¼ cup bacon fat, melted
- 4 garlic cloves, coarsely chopped (optional)

Instructions

1. Turn the cooker on High. Add onion and bacon into the cooker and cook, uncovered, until the fat has melted off the bacon.

2. Layer the cabbage pieces on top of the bacon-onion mixture.
3. Pour in the broth and add salt to taste.
4. Let the ingredients cook for an hour on High.
5. Stir the ingredients and continue cooking on High for no more than 4 hours.
6. Once done, drizzle some vinegar overtop and season with salt & pepper.
7. The cabbage is delicious served hot, and even better reheated the next day!

Nutrition Value: Protein: 1.77 g, Fat: 5.07g, Carbohydrate: 14.24g, Fiber: 4.1 g **Total Calories:** 108

19. Scrumptious Chicken Bacon Chowder

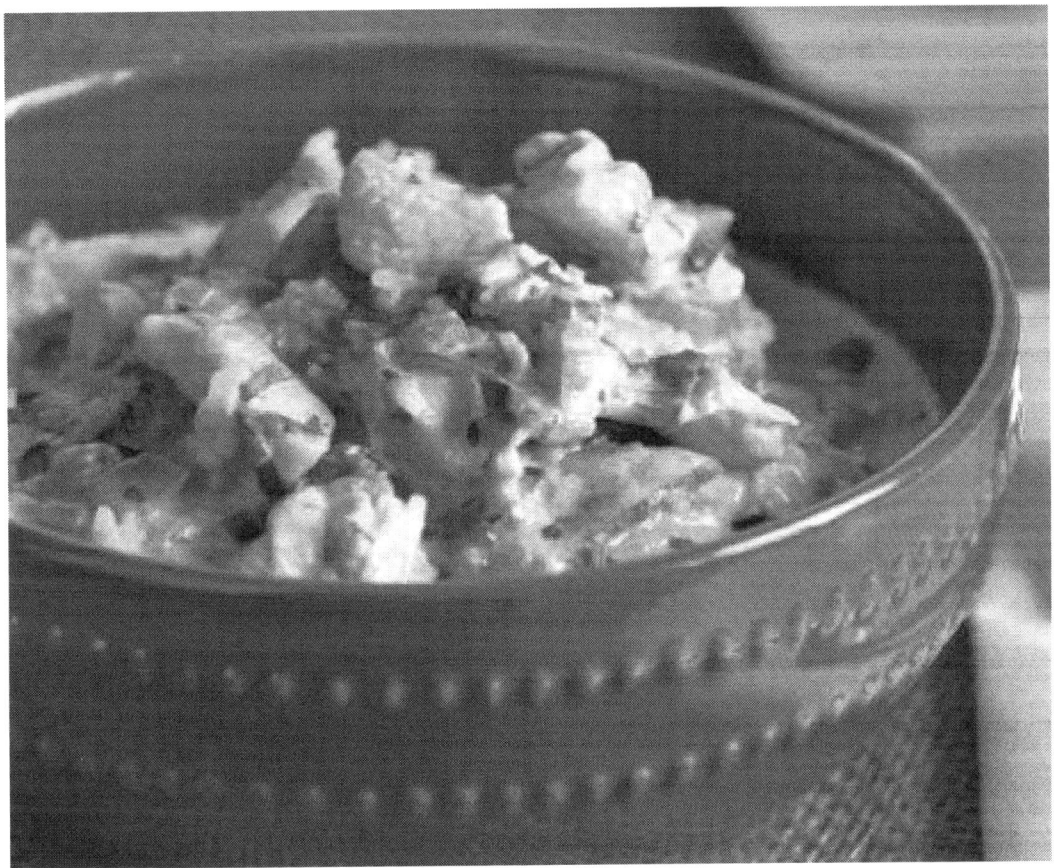

Ingredients

- 1 tsp dried thyme
- 1 tsp. black pepper
- 1 lb. bacon, cooked until crisp and crumbled
- 1 tsp. sea salt
- 8 oz. cream cheese
- 1 medium sweet onion, thinly sliced
- 1 lb. chicken breasts or thighs
- 1 cup heavy cream

- 2 ribs celery, diced
- 1 tsp. garlic powder
- 2 cups chicken stock, divided
- 1 small leek, cleaned, trimmed and sliced
- 6 mushrooms, sliced
- 1 shallot, finely chopped
- 4 cloves garlic, minced
- 4 tbsp. butter, divided

Instructions

1. Turn the cooker on Low. Add the leeks, black pepper, mushrooms, onions, 1 cup chicken stock, sea salt, 2 tbsp. butter, shallot, celery and garlic into the cooker and stir to combine. Cover and cook for about 30 mins.
2. Heat 2 tbsp. butter in a frying pan over medium heat and pan-sear the chicken breasts until browned on both sides. Set aside.
3. Add the remaining 1 cup of chicken stock to the slow cooker. Add the thyme, heavy cream, cream cheese, and garlic powder into the slow cooker. Carefully stir the ingredients.
4. After finely dicing the chicken, put it into the cooker with the bacon. Cook for 6-8 hours.

Nutrition Value: Protein: 21 g, Fat: 28 g, Carbohydrate: 6g, Fiber: 1 g
Total Calories: 355

20. Slow Cooker Jerk Chicken

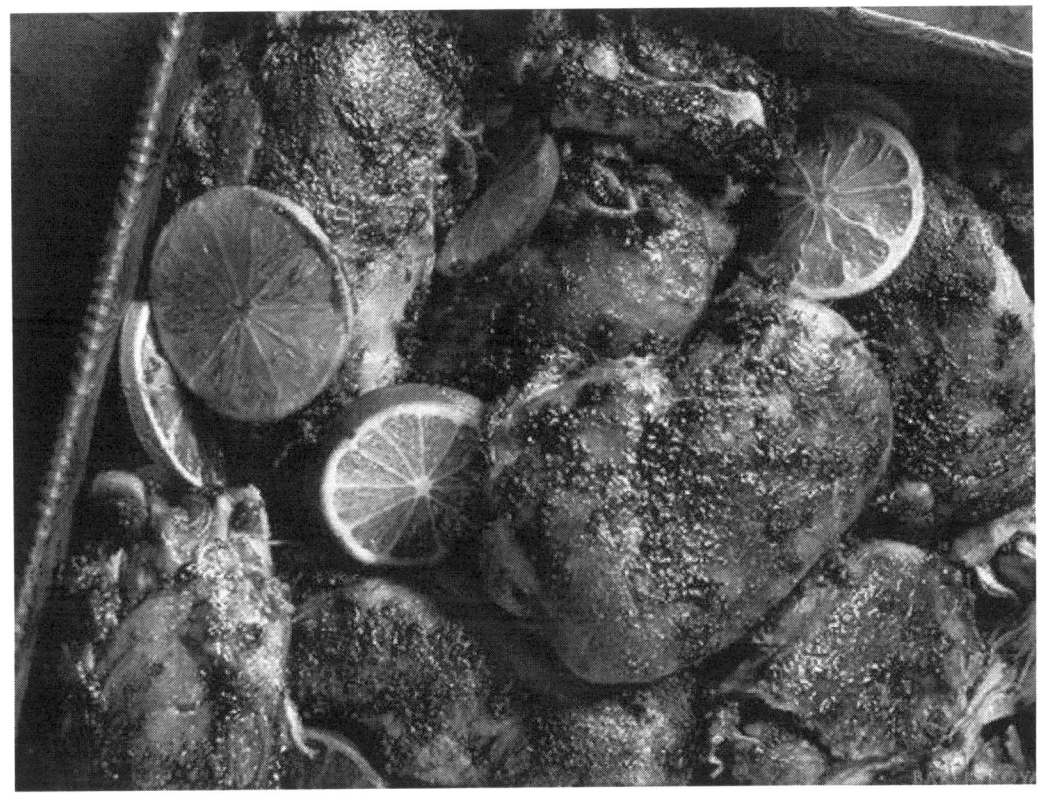

Ingredients

- 4 pounds bone-in, skin-on chicken pieces (split breasts, thighs)
- lime wedges for serving
- 2 tsp allspice
- 3 garlic cloves, peeled
- 1/4 teaspoon cardamom
- 1/4 cup vegetable oil
- 1 (1-inch) fresh ginger, peeled and sliced 1/4 inch thick
- 2 Tbsp. molasses
- 1 Tbsp. thyme
- 8 scallions, chopped coarse

- 1 teaspoon coarse salt
- 2 habanero chilies, stemmed and seeded

Instructions:

1. In a food processor, blend the cardamom, oil, ginger, molasses, scallion, garlic, habaneros, thyme, allspice, and salt. Pour the mixture into the slow cooker. Turn the slow cooker on High.
2. Coat chicken with scallion mixture and cook in the slow cooker, at least 5 minutes per side.
3. Cover and cook the chicken on Low for 5-6 hours.

Nutrition Value: Protein: 34.5 g, Fat: 11.5 g, Carbohydrate: 9.3 g, Fiber: 0.5 g **Total Calories:** 343.4

21. Slow Cooker Frittata

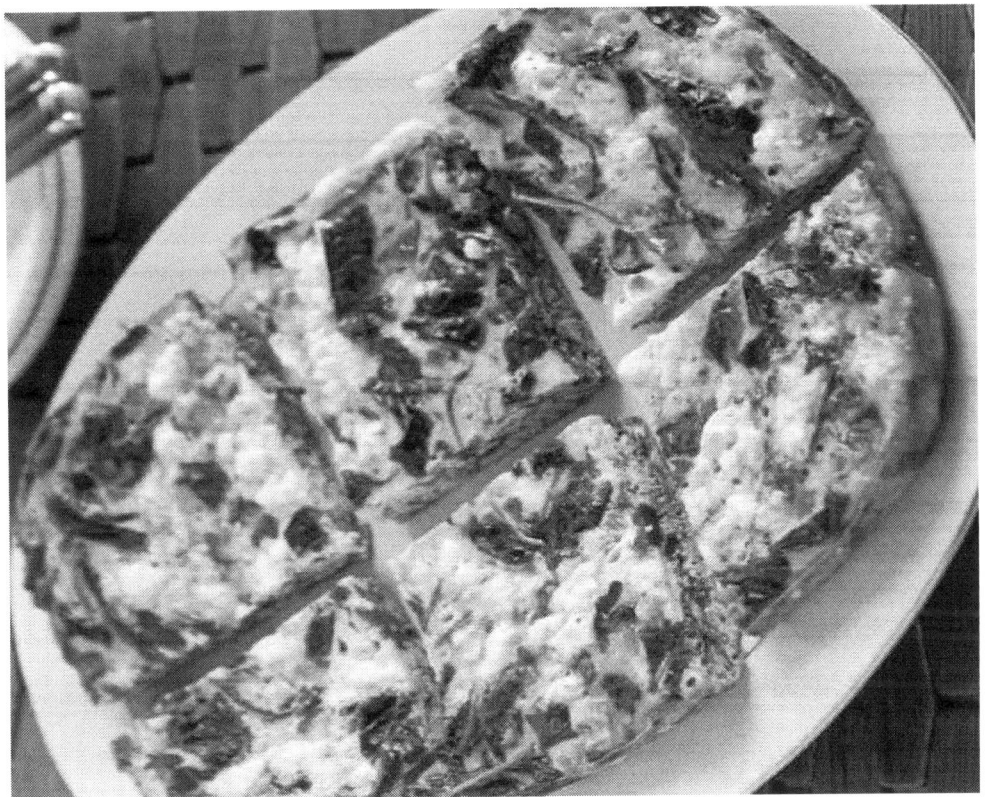

Ingredients

- 1/2 tsp Spike Seasoning
- 4-5 oz. crumbled Feta
- 8 oz. fresh kale, de-stemmed and chopped
- 6 oz. roasted red pepper
- non-stick spray or oil
- 8 eggs, well beaten
- 1/4 cup sliced green onion
- 1 - 2 tsp olive oil
- fresh-ground black pepper

Instructions

1. Heat the oil in a frying pan over medium heat and sauté the kale for 3-4 minutes.
2. Add the kale eggs, green onion and red pepper to the slow cooker and season with Spike Seasoning.
3. Sprinkle the feta overtop and cook on Low for 2 - 3 hours.

Nutrition Value: Protein: 26 g, Fat: 47 g, Carbohydrate: 11 g, Fiber: 1 g **Total Calories:** 590

22. Tasty Tarragon Lamb Shanks with Cannellini Beans

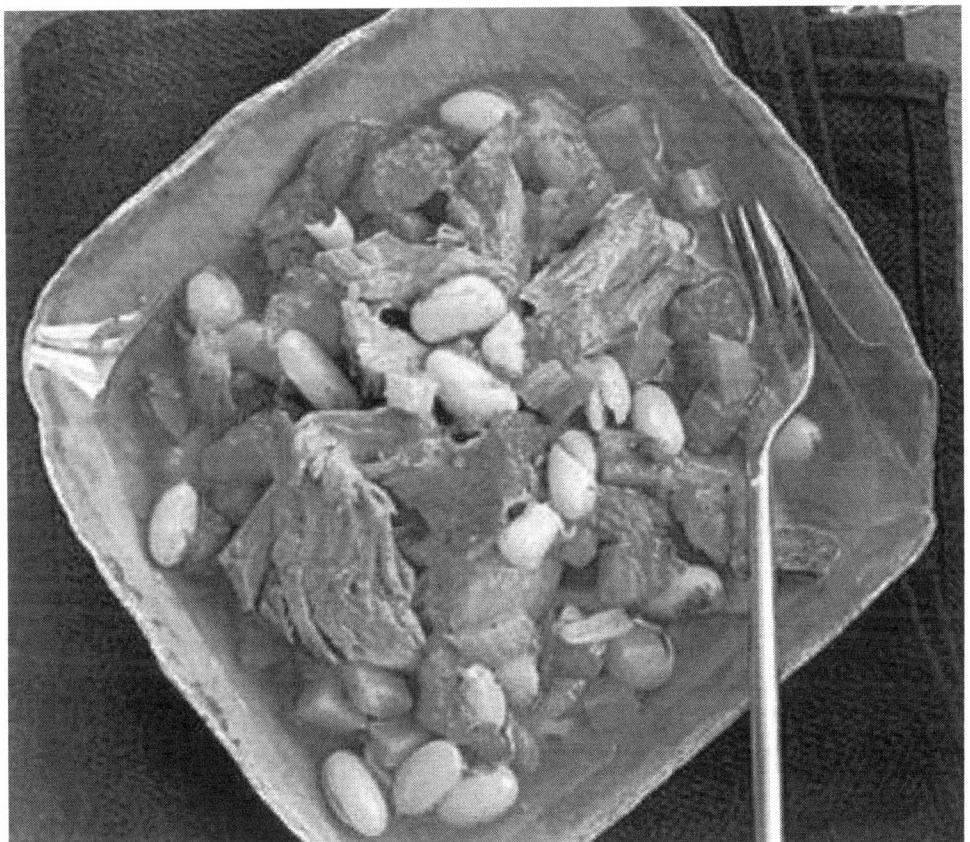

Ingredients

- 4 bone-in lamb shanks
- 1/4 tsp freshly ground black pepper
- 1 28-oz. can diced tomatoes
- 3/4 cup chopped celery
- 1 cup chopped onion
- 2 tsp dried tarragon
- 1 1/2 cups diced peeled carrot
- 1/2 tsp salt

- 1 19-oz can cannellini beans

Instructions

1. Place beans, tarragon, salt, tomatoes and pepper in the slow cooker. Position the lamb shanks among the mixture and cook on Low for 4-6 hours.
2. Remove the lamb shanks to a plate and remove the bones.
3. Spoon the bean mixture into a serving dish and top with the lamb shanks.

Nutrition Value: Protein: 36 g, Fat: 21 g, Carbohydrate: 9 g, Fiber: 7 g
Total Calories: 470

23. Delightful Carnitas & Paleo Nachos

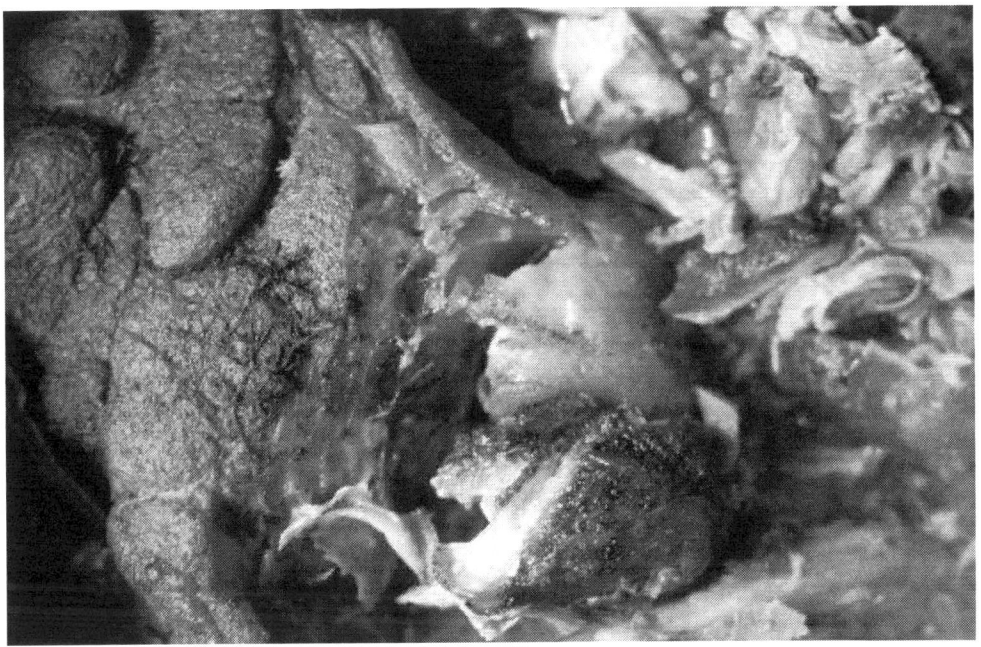

Ingredients

- 1 cup chicken broth or stock
- olive oil for frying
- 4 bay leaves
- 1.5 Tbsp. fresh thyme leaves
- 2-3 lb. pork shoulder
- sea salt and pepper

Instructions:

1. Rub the pork shoulder with salt and pepper. Heat the olive oil in a medium frying pan over medium-high heat and brown on all sides.

2. Place the bay leaves, pork, thyme and broth in the slow cooker.
3. Cook for 8-12 hours on Low.
4. Shred the meat with two forks and serve.

Nutrition Value: Protein: 35 g, Fat: 63 g, Carbohydrate: 37 g, Fiber: 16 g **Total Calories:** 1,080

24. Chicken Fajita Soup

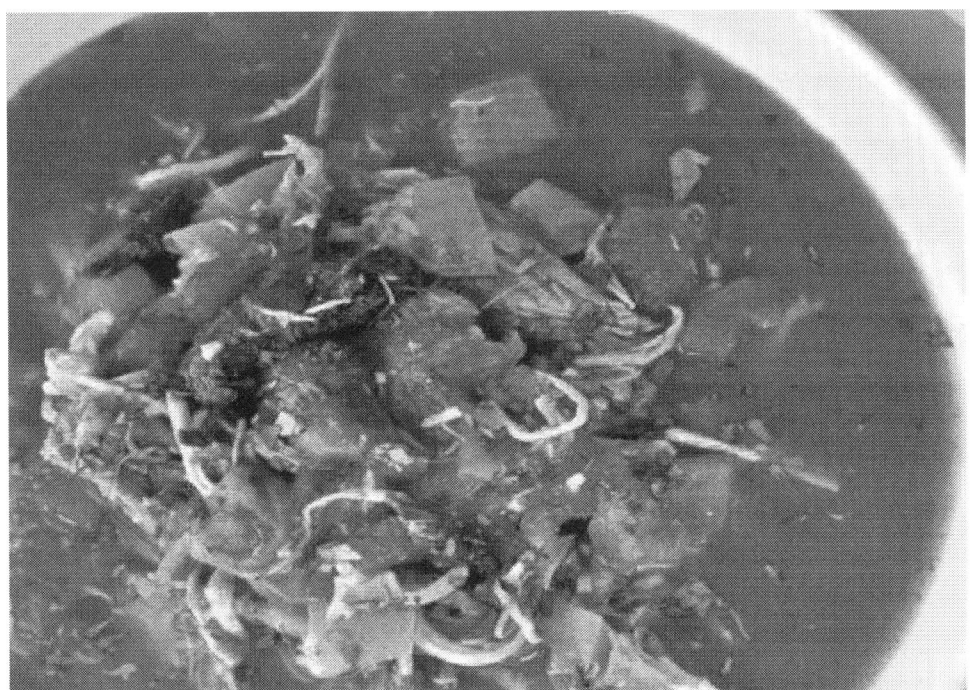

Ingredients

- 2 Tbsp. Taco Seasoning
- 2 large cloves garlic, minced
- 16 oz. chicken stock
- Salt more to taste
- 7.5-oz. can diced tomatoes
- 1 small onion, diced
- 1 Tbsp. fresh cilantro, chopped
- 1- 1/2 lbs. chicken breast
- 3 oz. mushrooms, thinly sliced
- 1 small yellow bell pepper, diced
- 1 small orange bell pepper, diced

Instructions:

1. Put all the ingredients; chicken, chicken stock, seasoning, cilantro and all vegetables in the slow cooker. Cook for 6 hours on Low.
2. Shred the chicken with two forks and cook for 1 additional hour.

Nutrition Value: Protein: 7 g, Fat: 9 g, Carbohydrate: 4 g, Fiber: 2 g
Total Calories: 200

25. Slow-Cooker Lemon and Olive Chicken

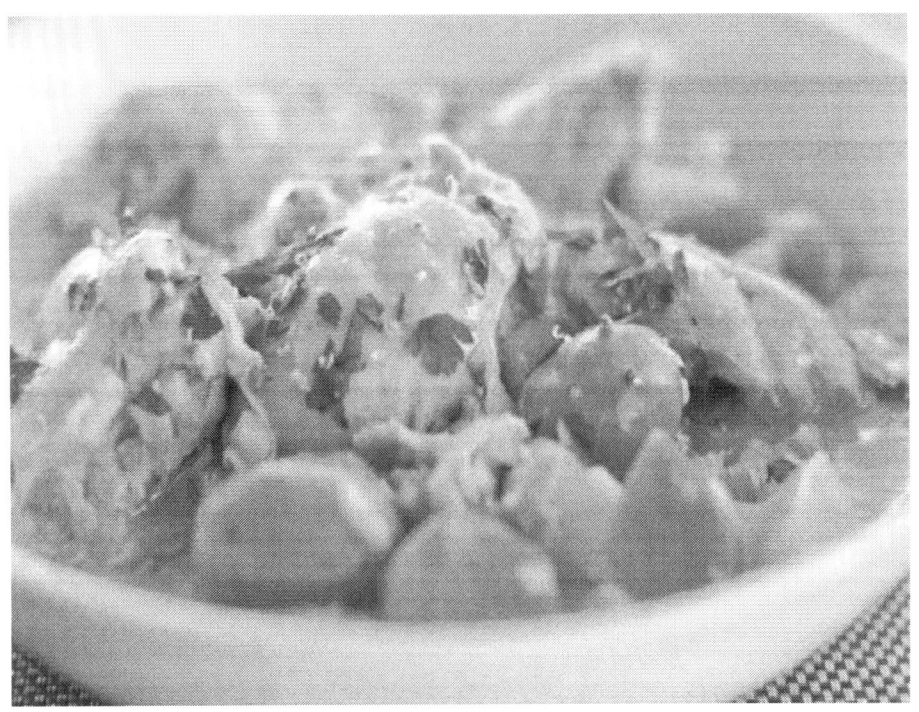

Ingredients

- 16 large stuffed green olives
- 1 Tbsp. lemon juice
- Grated zest of 1 lemon
- 2 ribs celery, chopped
- 4 cloves garlic, crushed
- 2 bay leaves
- ¼ cup all-purpose flour
- 1 onion, chopped
- 1 bulb fennel, cored and chopped
- 12 boneless skinless chicken thighs
- ¾ cup chicken broth
- ½ cup chopped fresh parsley
- ½ tsp. dried oregano

- Salt and pepper to taste
- 2 carrots, chopped

Instructions

1. Put all ingredients except flour and lemon juice in cooker and let it look for 5-6 hours on medium flame. Leave some herbs for garnishing.
2. Add in the flour with water and lemon juice for flavor. Let it cook in for further 15 minutes.
3. Add the garnishing and serve.

Nutrition Value: Protein: 18 g, Fat: 17 g, Carbohydrate: 10 g, Fiber: 32 g **Total Calories:** 176

26. Satisfying Pork Stew

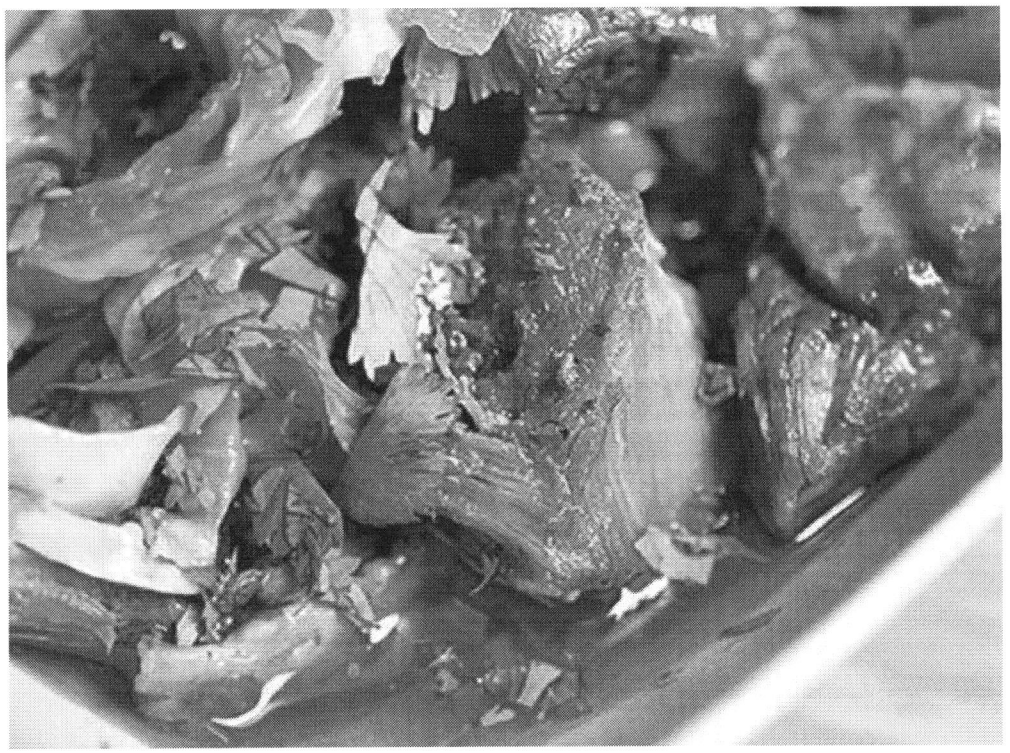

Ingredients

- 1 small onion, thinly sliced
- ½ small cabbage, cut into 4 wedges
- 3 cloves of garlic, smashed
- ¼ pound baby carrots
- 1 ½ pounds of pork shoulder, cut into 1-inch cubes
- ½ Tbsp. of your favorite seasoning blend
- ½ Tbsp. fish sauce
- ½ low-carb marinara sauce
- ½ Tbsp. vinegar
- Salt and pepper to taste

Instructions

1. Slice the carrots, onions and garlic and place in the cooker.
2. Season the beef with your favorite seasoning and layer the pork cubes over the vegetables in the slow cooker.
3. Add the cabbage wedges and top with the marinara sauce
4. Let cook 8-10 hours on Low. Season with salt, pepper, vinegar and herbs before serving.

Nutrition Value: Protein: 24 g, Fat: 7 g, Carbohydrate: 2 g, Fiber: 3 g
Total Calories: 272

27. Low-carb Slow-cooked Pizza

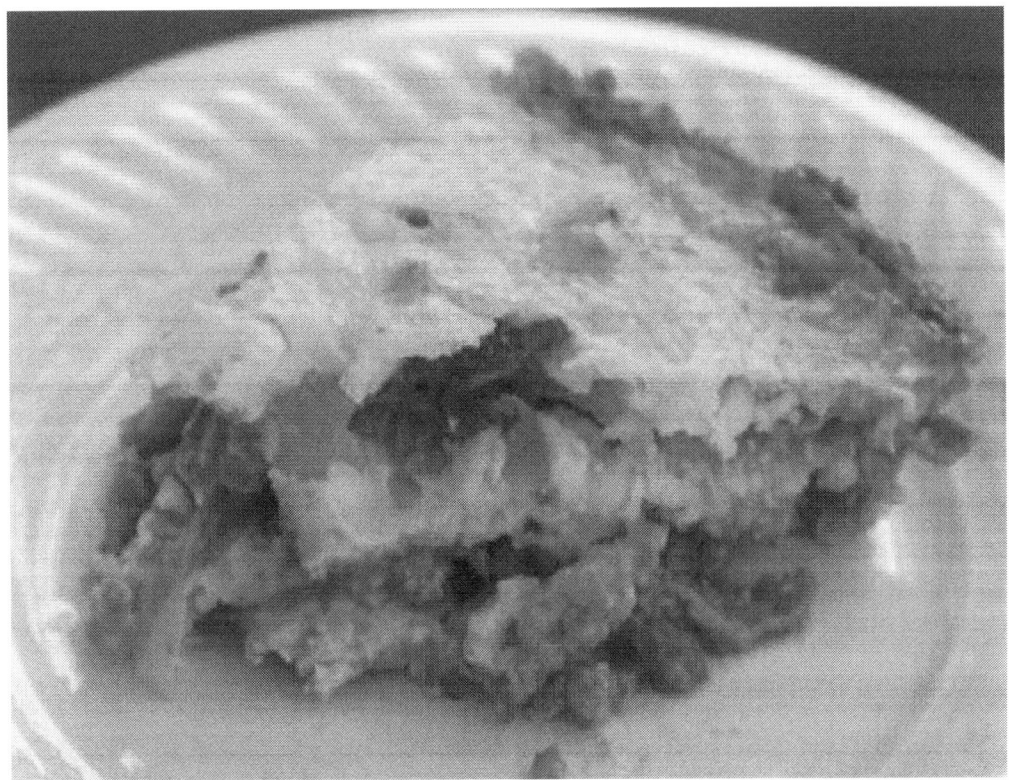

Ingredients

- ¾ lb. ground beef, cooked
- 3/4 lb. Italian sausage, cooked
- 3 cups mozzarella cheese, shredded
- 16 slices of low-carb pepperoni
- 1 15-oz. can pizza sauce
- 3 cups fresh spinach
- Any favorite topping like olives, mushrooms or herbs

Instructions

1. Slice the sausage, chop the onions and combine them with the pizza sauce. Divide the mixture in half and put one half into the slow cooker
2. Layer half of the fresh spinach on top of the sauce mixture
3. Layer half of the pepperoni and the remaining toppings on top.
4. Top with half of the cheese.
5. Repeat layers and cook for 6 hours. Let cool slightly before cutting and serving.

Nutrition Value: Protein: 14.3 g, Fat: 11.9 g, Carbohydrate: 5.4 g, Fiber: 0.5 g **Total Calories:** 186.4

28. Easy Italian Zucchini Meatloaf

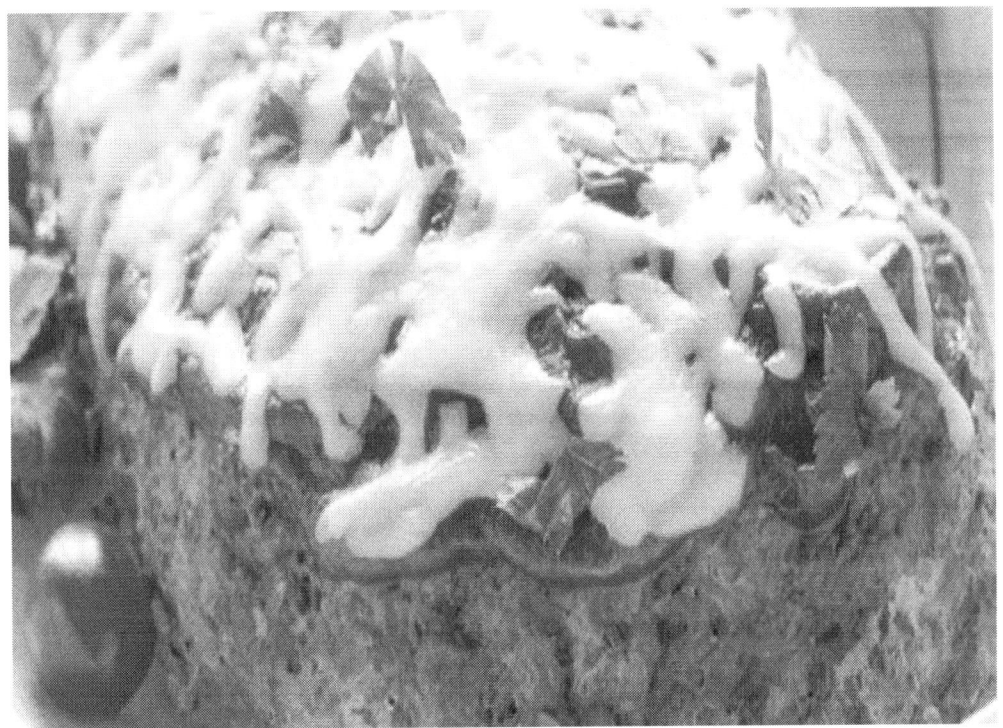

Ingredients

- 2 lbs. extra lean ground beef
- 2 large eggs
- 1 cup shredded zucchini
- 1/2 cup grated Parmesan cheese
- 1/2 cup finely chopped parsley
- 4 crushed garlic cloves
- 2 tbsp. balsamic vinegar
- 1 tbsp. dry oregano
- 2 tbsp. minced dry onion or onion powder
- Salt to taste

- 1/2 tsp ground black pepper
- Cooking coconut oil spray

Instructions

1. Place all the ingredients in a large bowl and mix thoroughly.
2. Prepare the slow cooker by lining with aluminum foil with flaps on the outside, to make it easier to remove the meatloaf later. Spray the lining with coconut oil spray.
3. Put the mixture in cooker. Cover and cook on Low for about 6 hours, or on High for 2-2.5 hours.

Nutrition Value: Protein: 20.7g, Fat: 9 g, Carbohydrate: 3.4 g, Fiber: 0.1 g **Total Calories:** 97.5

29. Hearty Beef Stew

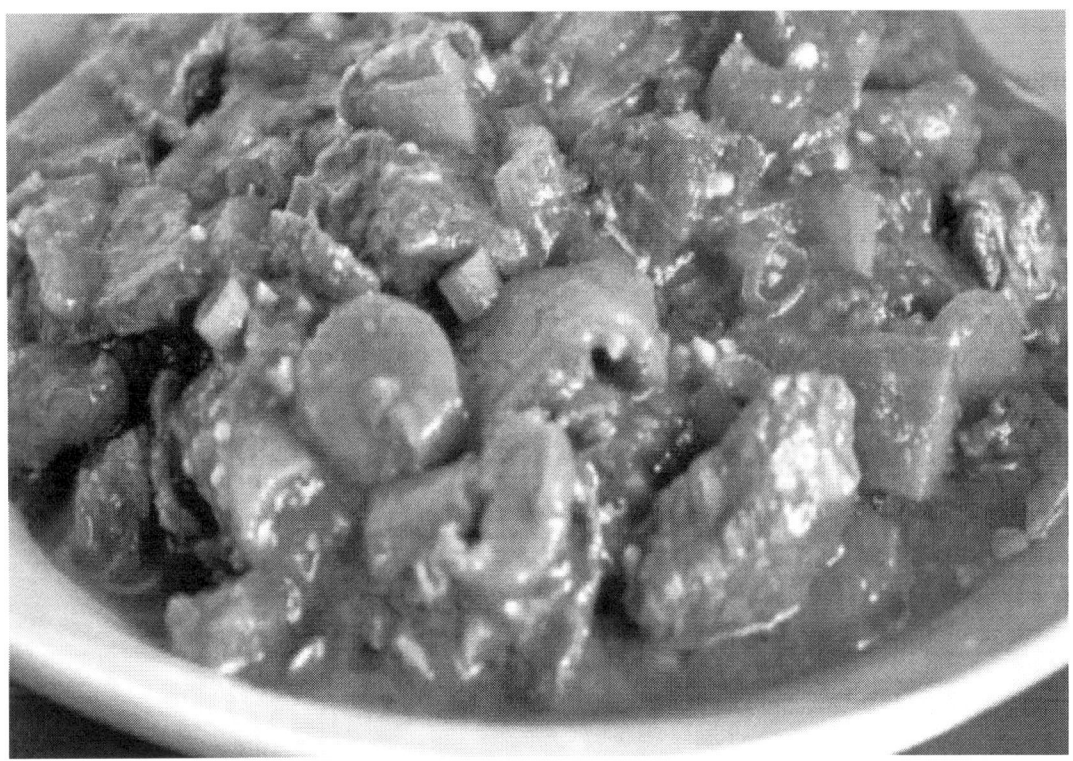

Ingredients
- 1 lbs. stewing beef
- 1.5   Tbsp. olive oil
- 1 cup beef stock
- 6 oz. cooked crisp bacon
- 7 oz. diced tomatoes
- 2 oz. chopped bell peppers
- 2 oz. sliced mushrooms
- 1 rib chopped celery
- 1 medium sized chopped carrot

- half a small onion, chopped
- 2 large cloves garlic, finely chopped
- 2 Tbsp. tomato paste
- 1 Tbsp. Worcestershire sauce
- sea salt to taste
- 1/2 tsp. black pepper
- 1 tsp. dried Oregano

Instructions
1. Prepare slow cooker on low heat setting.
2. In a large skillet over high heat, sear the beef on both sides.
3. Place all the ingredients and the seared beef in the slow cooker.
4. Cover and cook on Low for 6-7 hours.

Nutrition Value: Protein: 22g, Fat: 15 g, Carbohydrate: 5 g, Fiber: 1 g
Total Calories: 235

30. Easy Slow-cooker Chicken Roast

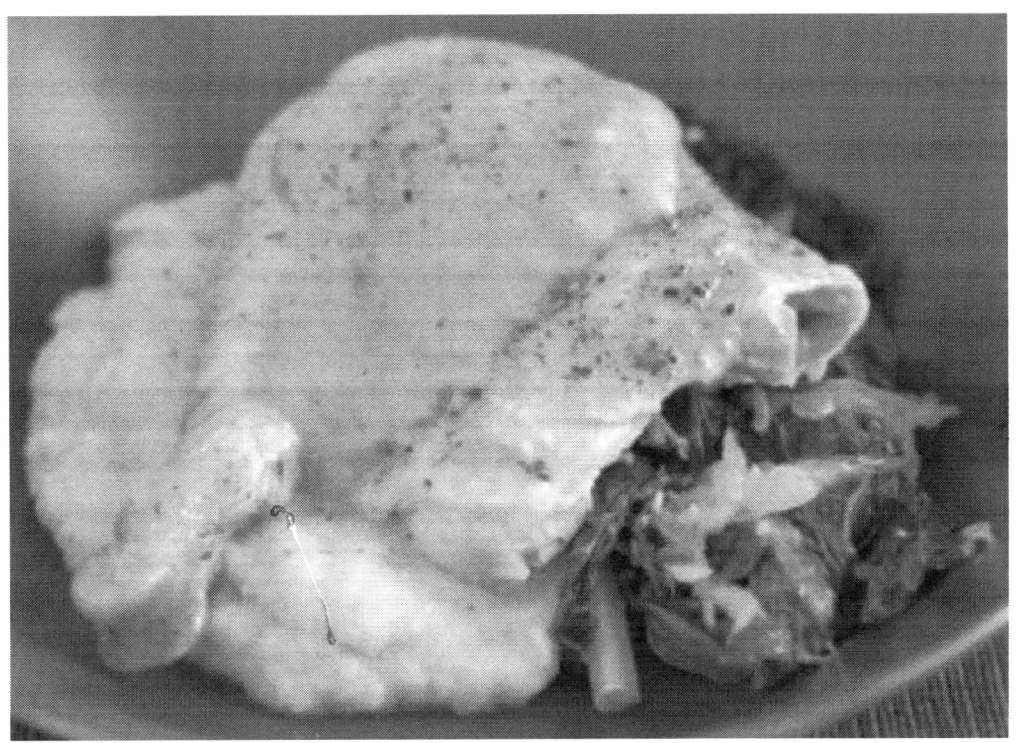

Ingredients
- 3-4 pound whole organic chicken
- 2 Tbsp. homemade ghee
- 2 medium sized chopped onions
- 1 clove of peeled garlic
- 1 tsp tomato paste
- ¼ cup chicken stock
- ¼ cup white wine
- 1 tbsp. freshly ground black pepper
- Kosher salt to taste
- 1 tsp dried mixed Italian herbs

Instructions

1. In a hot cast iron pan, sauté all the vegetables in ghee. Add the tomato paste and season with salt and pepper. Cook for 5-7 minutes until the vegetables are slightly softened.
2. Deglaze the pan with wine or chicken stock. Add all the vegetables into the slow cooker. Season the chicken with salt and pepper and place it breast side down in the slow cooker.
3. Cook the chicken for 3-4 hours on Low.

Nutrition Value: Protein: 30.1 g, Fat: 4.1 g, Carbohydrate: 1.4 g, Fiber: 0.6 g **Total Calories:** 169.6

FAQs

•Can I drink alcohol or coffee on the Atkins Diet?

You may consume a limited amount of alcohol, but it is not recommended as alcohol consumption will likely interfere with your goal of losing weight. Refraining from consuming alcohol in the beginning stages of the Atkins diet is really helpful and the results are significant. However, in the later stages of the Atkins diet, you can reintroduce alcohol. It is suggested to avoid mixing the alcohol with anything; instead, take it neat. This will make it easier to calculate your Net Carbs intake.

•Can you drink soda and juices on the Atkins Diet?

Consumption of artificial sweeteners like soda and juices is a sensitive matter. Different people respond differently to soda intake, and artificial sweeteners can slow the progress of weight loss. If you drink soda, it should be caffeine-free. Aspartame is not allowed because it may interfere with your weight loss goals, and many diet sodas contain aspartame. Soda that contains sucralose and stevia are allowed in the Atkins Diet, but excessive intake of these beverages can halt your weight loss. According to the Atkins website, "one serving of sweetener is equivalent to 3 tsp. of powdered sucralose or stevia, two packets of sucralose or stevia, or 12 oz. of allowed diet soda."

•How much weight can I lose by following the Atkins Diet?

According to Dr. Atkins, "You can expect to lose 6-10 lbs. in the first two weeks of Induction, which should slow to 1-3 lbs. a week once you enter the Ongoing Weight Loss Phase." Throughout the Pre-maintenance phase, one can lose up to 1 lb. a week.

- **Is this diet suitable for PCOS patients?**

The major symptom of PCOS is an irregular menstrual cycle, or no menstruation at all. Maintaining a proper diet and staying active can help you to recover from PCOS. The Atkins Diet is based on a low intake of sugar and carbohydrates, which is perfect for PCOS patients. A PCOS patient may also follow a vegan version of the Atkins Diet. This can also prevent chronic diseases.

- **Is this diet suitable for diabetics?**

The Atkins theory suggests that high sugar consumption actually promotes the unnecessary production of insulin in the body. This in return, makes our body less receptive to insulin. When our body fails to respond to insulin, many chronic diseases like diabetes can result. Lowering one's carbohydrate intake can prevent these chronic diseases, since it will result in fewer blood-sugar spikes throughout the day. However, please consult with your doctor before making any changes to your treatment plan or medication.

- **Is the Atkins Diet compatible with veganism?**

It is a misconception that a vegan can't follow the Atkins Diet. The Atkins Diet simply implements a lower consumption of carbohydrates and sugar. It is not mandatory to eat meat or animal products, so other than reducing carbohydrate and sugar intake, a vegan diet would not be affected by following Atkins.

- **How can I ensure a nutritionally balanced diet when on Atkins?**

The Atkins Diet is based on a diversity of food. The Atkins Diet recommends consuming vegetables, dairy products, soy, legumes, berries and any other foods that have a low carbohydrate content and high fiber- plus- fat content. Therefore, ordinary nutritional recommendations still apply; whether you follow the Canadian Food

Guide (food pyramid) or a macro diet (tracking and balancing intake of protein, fat and carbohydrates), Atkins is very compatible with a nutritionally balanced diet.

Conclusion

Atkins Diet isn't like most temporary, quick-fix diet plans. Atkins is a lifestyle; a healthy one. The detailed plan, the variety of allowed foods and the simplicity of the slow-cooking method make the Atkins Diet a practical approach for weight loss and weight maintenance.

It is true, the journey won't be easy, but it is do-able. All you need is motivation and willpower to implement the diet; once you start to see the changes you're looking for, you will find motivation all on your own. Soon you'll fulfill your goals and look your best with your healthy body!

Made in the USA
Middletown, DE
21 January 2018